HOSPITAL CARE OF CHILDREN AND YOUTH

1986 EDITION

Author: Committee on Hospital Care
American Academy of Pediatrics
Joseph M. Garfunkel, M.D., Consulting Editor
Hugh E. Evans, M.D., Editor

American Academy of Pediatrics
P.O. Box 927, 141 Northwest Point Boulevard
Elk Grove Village, Illinois 60007

Committee on Hospital Care

Hugh E. Evans, M.D., Chairman 1985-
Paul S. Bergeson, M.D., Chairman 1981-1985

Alfred Amler, M.D.
Arnold Anderson, M.D.
Fred T. Brown, M.D.
Martha Bushore, M.D.
James C. Cravens, M.D.
David L. Dudgeon, M.D.
Harvey Gold, M.D.

Michael A. Hogan, M.D.
Hugh Lynn, M.D.
Charles Lockhart, M.D.
James E. Shira, M.D.
Theodore Striker, M.D.
Willis Wingert, M.D.

Consultant

Joseph Garfunkel, M.D., Consulting Editor

Liaisons

James W. Dilley, M.D., Joint Commission on Accreditation
of Hospitals
Paul Donnelly, American Hospital Association
Hervy B. Kornegay, M.D., American Academy of Family
Physicians
H.W. Maysent, American Hospital Association
Fred Marienau, M.D., American Academy of Family
Physicians
Russell C. Raphaely, M.D., AAP Section on Critical Care
Medicine
James Robert, M.D., Joint Commission on Accreditation of
Hospitals
Barbara-Jeanne Seabury, Association for the Care of
Children's Health
Donald E. Widmann, M.D., Joint Commission on
Accreditation of Hospitals

Library of Congress Catalog No. 78-53173

ISBN 0-910761-09-4

Quantity prices on request. Address all inquiries to:
American Academy of Pediatrics, P.O. Box 927, 141 Northwest Point
Boulevard, Elk Grove Village, Illinois 60007
©1986 by the American Academy of Pediatrics. All rights reserved.
Printed in the United States of America

Introduction

Never in the history of pediatrics have there been so many extraordinary demands on all health care providers involved in the hospital care of children and youth. There have been developments in many areas, including medical technology, regionalization, financing and cost containment, hospital management, architecture, and attention to the emotional needs of hospitalized children. It is important, therefore, that a resource be available which compiles recent and useful material to expedite the work of health care professionals, planners, and agency officials. A concerted attempt has been made in *Hospital Care of Children and Youth, 1986* to fulfill this need by providing a general philosophy of child care, a concise and useful text, an extended bibliography, and a set of appendices. The Committee on Hospital Care hopes that the publication of this manual will result in improved care to children, and this hope is the ultimate motivation for the expenditure of the considerable effort and expense involved in its production.

Hospital Care of Children and Youth, 1986 should be viewed as a collection of suggestions; no attempt has been made to define standards. Indeed, because of the rapid evolution in the nature of hospital care, the ideas in this manual should be used in a flexible fashion and modified to fit local circumstances and inevitable changes in the practice of medicine. The Committee acknowledges that many health care concepts have escaped inclusion and that this manual is not all-inclusive in nature. Rapidly changing strategies designed to contain medical costs, such as diagnosis related groups (DRG's) and prospective reimbursement plans, may profoundly change the pattern of hospital use and, ultimately, of office practice. The impact of "Baby Doe" legislation and federal administrative action likewise will be of great significance. However, these developments are too fluid to include in a manual of this type. The professional literature and lay press undoubtedly will cover these issues in great detail over the coming years.

Paul S. Bergeson, M.D., Chairman 1981-1985
Hugh E. Evans, M.D., Chairman 1985-
Joseph M. Garfunkel, M.D., Consulting Editor

Acknowledgment

The Committee is profoundly grateful to a variety of consultants who have unselfishly provided many hours and considerable skills to the writing of the individual chapters of *Hospital Care of Children and Youth, 1986*.

The Committee acknowledges the following individuals for the contributions they have made to this manual:

Mary Layne Ahern, Esq., Chicago, Illinois
Alfred V. Amler, M.D., New York, New York
Laura Borden, R.N., B.S.N., Knoxville, Tennessee
George M. Bright, M.D., Richmond, Virginia
Deal Chandler Brooks, M.A., Chicago, Illinois
L. Joseph Butterfield, M.D., Denver, Colorado
Daniel N. Davidow, M.D., Richmond, Virginia
Paul L. Donnelly, Spokane, Washington
John P. Dorst, M.D., Baltimore, Maryland
Blaise E. Favara, M.D., Halifax, Nova Scotia, Canada
Donald C. Fischer, M.D.
Donald Frank, M.D., Cincinnati, Ohio
Stanford B. Friedman, M.D., Baltimore, Maryland
Robert H. Gregg, M.D., Hartford, Connecticut
Alvin Hackel, M.D., Palo Alto, California
Herman A. Hein, M.D., Iowa City, Iowa
Peter R. Holbrook, M.D., Washington, D.C.
John Jeffries, M.H.A., Buffalo, New York
Arlene Kiely, R.N., Washington, D.C.
Hugh B. Lynn, M.D., Middleburg, Virginia
Marvin I. Mones, M.D., Silver Spring, Maryland
Gerald Nathenson, M.D., Bronx, New York
Charlotte G. Neumann, M.D., M.P.H., Los Angeles, California
Stephen S. Perry, Jr.
Emma Plank, M.A., Vienna, Austria
Joseph E. Simon, M.D., Marietta, Georgia
E. Ide Smith, M.D., Oklahoma City, Oklahoma
Marian Susuki, B.A., R.D., Los Angeles, California
Lawrence Taft, M.D., New Brunswick, New Jersey
William P. Tunell, M.D., Tulsa, Oklahoma
Michael D. Tyne, Columbus, Ohio
Philip D. Walson, M.D., Columbus, Ohio
William W. Waring, M.D., New Orleans, Louisiana
Irvin G. Wilmot
Jerriann M. Wilson, M.Ed., Baltimore, Maryland
Willis A. Wingert, M.D., Los Angeles, California

Contents

Chapter 1

COMMUNITY PLANNING FOR HOSPITAL CARE

Community hospitals, regardless of size, usually have included a pediatric unit. It has been typical of family physicians and pediatricians to hospitalize children at community hospitals for such surgical procedures as tonsillectomy, adenoidectomy, or appendectomy, and for such medical problems as infections or gastrointestinal diseases, especially those associated with high fever and/or fluid loss.

The pattern of care provided for children has changed during the past 10 years. Some surgical procedures, such as tonsillectomies and cystoscopies, are performed less often. A trend toward "one-day stay" or ambulatory surgery has emerged. Board-certified or qualified pediatric surgeons are increasingly available in both university centers and community hospitals. Viral illnesses and the usually benign nature of most fevers are now better understood. Even moderately severe gastroenteritis usually can be controlled by judicious use of oral fluids. Bacterial infections formerly managed in the hospital now are commonly treated on an outpatient basis. Hence, the need for pediatric departments in small community hospitals is much less apparent than in the past.

A growing public awareness of the specialized needs of sick children likewise militates against their care in small hospitals. Physicians with minimal training and/or experience in dealing with diseases of childhood are unwilling to risk an untoward result and the likelihood of malpractice litigation. Thus, it seems likely that more children in the future will receive hospital care in a facility designed to meet their needs and by physicians trained in pediatric medicine and surgery. In rural and underserved areas, specialized hospital care for children may be provided mainly on a regional basis.

Despite the many reasons to centralize hospital care of children in specialized facilities, the primary care providers for many children will continue to be local physicians, either pediatricians or family physicians. These physicians are the primary access point into any regionalized care network, and they must have ample basic input in formulating plans for the hospital needs of their child patients.

Planning for Hospital Care in a Regionalized System

Care for the Future: Regionalization

Provision of care matched to need, or regionalization, has proved conducive to a beneficial outcome for perinatal patients in this country.[1,2] The concept of regionalization is the product not of genius but of necessity. As techniques of care improve and financial resources shrink, the concept of regionalization probably will be strengthened.

DRG's and HMO's

Two recent developments have significant potential impact on provision of health care for children, namely, payment mechanisms based on diagnosis related groups (DRG's) and the increased number of health maintenance organizations (HMO's). The possible effects are only speculative, but it is likely that the DRG payment mechanism will have an impact on case mixture, length of stay, and range of services offered. However, HMO's could have an opposite effect. Because referral of patients outside the HMO may be costly to the group, there may be a reluctance to refer patients, and a tendency to manage many patients locally may emerge.

Because profitability under the DRG system will be predicated on the same basis as under HMO's (namely, the shortest hospital stay incorporating the fewest tests and the lowest cost), it is possible that both DRG's and HMO's may compromise quality of care. However, prime consideration must be given to providing the best care for the hospitalized child.

The Planning Process

Initial planning for hospital care of children should be

based on regional as well as local evaluation of patient needs. Effective local planning can evolve after a general plan for the region has been developed.

The major goal of regional planning is to offer each child in the region the opportunity to receive modern care appropriately matched to the complexity of the illness. Some regions will contain facilities representative of all three levels of care (refer to Addendum on levels of care). The planning challenge is one of cooperative classification of facilities, acceptance of designation, provision of transport services, and maintenance of the system through peer-directed review and education.

Participation in the regional planning process should come from all the involved levels of care. Planning cannot begin until regional boundaries have been defined. Some regions may not have tertiary care centers *per se* and should develop cooperative agreements with tertiary care centers outside the region. In some regions, Level II facilities may be nonexistent or underrepresented, and illnesses of moderate complexity that ordinarily could be managed in such centers may require referral to a tertiary care center. Because of recognized differences among regions, planners are cautioned to give prime consideration to the special needs of their region rather than attempt to transform the region according to prescribed models.

Even though formal regionalized systems of care may not have existed previously, established patterns of referral of sick children probably will have been in effect for some time. A survey of referral practices among primary care physicians in the region will determine the naturally occurring referral patterns. If these patterns are respected rather than attempting to impose a totally different system, primary care givers undoubtedly will cooperate more readily. In general, strengthening existing referral systems rather than redesigning them will help to avoid unnecessary jurisdictional disputes.

Suggestions for regional planning for hospital care of children given in this chapter are based on considerations of needs of children in the immediate future. The basis for this material is the experience gained in the development of a regional system of perinatal health care for the state of Iowa.[3-5] Although specific problems of pregnant women and sick neonates are different from those of sick children, the basic approach to systems development should be similar.

Development of the Plan

Initiating the Process

The regional plan should serve the interests of all children in the region. It is important that individuals representative of the various locales and levels of care have an opportunity to influence the design of the plan. A regional advisory committee should be developed and should consist of a broad representation from consumer and provider groups. Requisites for representation may vary among regions, but a representative group may include the following:
- pediatricians (general and subspecialists), including osteopathic physicians;
- pediatric surgeons, surgical subspecialists, including osteopathic physicians and anesthesiologists;
- pediatric nurses;
- family physicians, including osteopathic physicians;
- social service representatives;
- parents;
- public health nursing representatives;
- hospital administrators;
- emergency medical services representatives (transport).

Initially, it is necessary to resolve the issue of leadership or responsibility for the regional system of care. Implementation of a regional plan probably fails more frequently because of a lack of responsible leadership with sufficient time and energy than because of inadequate plan design. Regardless of the excellence of the plan, problems will arise. Accordingly, an individual or small committee should be designated as having the responsibility to make decisions. Because the tertiary care center will be the hub of regional activities, it is important that the regional director be able to work harmoniously with the pediatric department chairperson.

The regional advisory committee will be responsible for the

development of a working document which will allow the process of determining regional needs. The advisory committee ultimately must determine the following:

1. number and type of facilities in the region;
2. types of providers associated with facilities;
3. time/distance factors in the region;
4. transport needs based on time/distance factors;
5. financial arrangements among institutions within the region, including cost of transport;
6. method of maintaining the system through peer review and education.

Determining Regional Needs

The regional director should select a team of providers experienced in child health care to begin a survey of the region. Hospitals in the region should be visited to determine the following:

1. size of facility;
2. adequacy of the facility;
3. number of types of providers on staff;
4. nature of patient population currently served;
5. regional referral area or pattern of referral;
6. distance from other facilities;
7. other obstacles impeding access to care.

The survey team should be capable of assessing the quality of care provided in the hospital. This information is helpful in determining the designated level of care as well as planning for future educational needs.

Planning the System

Designation of Centers

On completion of the regional survey, the advisory committee and the survey team can begin the process of designation of levels of care. Because of the wide variation of patient needs, provider skills, and types of facilities among regions, it is not feasible to offer guidelines for center designation in this manual. The important issue is to develop a system that is practical and feasible for the region. Whether or not this system conforms to prescribed models should be of little concern.

Transport System

A properly functioning regional system of care for children must provide appropriate transport capability. Transport requirements will vary according to climate, geography, and population density. The regional survey should provide specific information about transport needs in the region. (See Chapter 18 for specific details of pediatric transport systems.)

Financial Considerations

The cost of developing and maintaining a regional system of care for children is a matter of public policy. Because regional systems of care are designed for the public good, government agencies responsible for public health in the area should provide financial support, but they should not necessarily be expected to fund the entire cost. Referral hospitals also benefit from these regional systems and may in some instances be asked to contribute to the costs.

An important consideration in regional planning is financial support for patient care. Financial considerations should never prevent a critically ill child from receiving care. However, they may delay referrals. Appropriate planning by hospital administrators, physicians, social welfare agencies, and emergency medical services (transport) representatives can prevent problems related to payment mechanisms.

Maintaining the System

Proper maintenance of a system of care is perhaps the most difficult facet of planning. It is relatively easy for a planning group to assemble a regional planning document. However, this document will be ineffective if proper maintenance of the system is not well developed. Specifically, maintenance involves the following:

1. Regular contact by tertiary care center providers with Level I and Level II counterparts—This can be accomplished by visits of tertiary care center personnel to referring facilities. These visits should focus on patient care activities, review of care practices, and provision of education pertinent to current or potential problems encountered in the hospital. The visits should be nonjudgmental in nature and conducted solely for the purpose of improving patient care. Even though medical records review may be used to determine educational needs, patient and physician identification should be avoided. These visits improve care by imparting current medical knowledge, and they remove emotional barriers to consultation and referral by allowing the individuals involved with patient care at the various levels of care to become acquainted with one another. Level II facilities that receive referrals should provide similar visits to their referring hospitals.

2. Provision of frequent communications regarding the status of patients referred—It is essential that referral centers provide follow-up data to local providers. Because the referring (or primary) physician must continue to deal with family members, accurate and timely information about the sick child is essential.

3. Return of patient to care of the referring physician—Physicians receiving referral patients should ensure that the patient returns to the care of the referring physician when his or her clinical condition permits. Parents may express a desire to continue care by physicians at the referral center. When this occurs and the child's clinical condition does not warrant it, the parents should be urged to return to the primary physician. If the parents persist, the referring physician should be informed personally of the parents' desires by the physician involved at the center.

4. Development of a central clearinghouse for problems related to children's care in the region—The regional director and survey-education team should be available at a central office location to deal with consultations and concerns relating to patient care and administrative problems within the region. Providers in the region must understand how and where concerns can be registered, and be assured that these concerns will receive prompt attention.

Addendum

Levels of Care

The Committee on Hospital Care recognizes the principle that delivery of child health care generally can be categorized into three levels, depending on the availability of personnel and facilities or equipment. The concept of regionalization of child health care includes the ability to transport children from one type of hospital to another when the need for a change in level of care becomes apparent. Similarly, within a given hospital, there may be separate or related facilities that provide different levels of care; this enables the hospital to provide care appropriate to the needs of children with a wide spectrum of medical or surgical problems. The following definitions are intended as guidelines for both individual hospital and regional planning.

Level I

Level I hospitals provide initial, tentative diagnosis and treatment, in either an ambulatory or inpatient setting, of a type commonly accomplished by a primary care physician. These hospitals also should provide immediate care and stabilization of pediatric patients with more severe problems while preparing them for transfer to a Level II or III hospital. Level I hospitals should have an established relationship with Level II and/or III hospitals to facilitate transfers of patients and to allow for educational support and consultation by the advanced level institutions. Most Level I hospitals will be in rural areas; little justification exists for a Level I pediatric unit in a metropolitan area.

Level II

Level II hospitals provide care at a level generally expected of a Board-certified or qualified pediatrician or similarly qualified specialist. Pediatric units of this type commonly are located in community hospitals and often have an association with a Level III hospital. The range of problems that can be managed adequately will vary with the availability of consultants and physical facilities but includes most illnesses of intermediate complexity. Other factors to be taken into account include climate, distance from more sophisticated facilities, the practicality and availability of transport mechanisms, and economic and family considerations. A Level II hospital may have Level III capabilities for some medical or surgical problems.

Level III

Level III hospitals provide definitive, comprehensive management of patients with complex and technologically demanding illnesses. Their capabilities must include the continuous availability of specialists, subspecialists, and appropriate support personnel as well as comprehensive, modern facilities and equipment. An inherent characteristic of Level III hospitals is the presence of educational and/or research programs.

Communication

The Level I, II, and III hospitals in any region should interrelate closely via continuing communication, referrals, and educational activities. Referral of patients among the three levels of care must depend on the clinical judgment of the patient's personal physician.

References

1. Hein, H.A.: Evaluation of a rural perinatal care system. Pediatrics, 66:540, 1980.
2. Committee on Fetus and Newborn and Committee on Obstetrics: Maternal and Fetal Medicine: Guidelines for Perinatal Care. Evanston, Illinois: American Academy of Pediatrics, and Washington, D.C.: American College of Obstetricians and Gynecologists, p. 7, 1983.

3. Hein, H.A., Christopher, C., and Ferguson, N.N.: Rural perinatology. Pediatrics, 55:769, 1975.
4. Hein, H.A.: Regionalization of perinatal care in rural areas based on the Iowa experience. Semin. Perinatol., 1:241, 1977.
5. Hein, H.A.: Common sense and health planning in rural areas. Perinatol. Neonatol., 6:65, September-October, 65, 1982.

Chapter 2

ADMINISTRATION

Organization

The administration of hospital services for children varies, depending on whether they are rendered in a children's hospital, in the pediatric unit of a general hospital, or in the pediatric service of a major teaching hospital. Other factors include the size of the department, the range of services offered, the socioeconomic spectrum represented, and the physical plant.

Overview

A table of organization—which clearly defines the interrelationships of the governing body, the administration, and the medical staff—should be developed.

In small or medium-sized hospitals, the administrator usually will be directly responsible to the governing body for all the hospital's activities, including those of the medical staff. In large general hospitals and many children's hospitals, a chief executive officer is accountable for all hospital affairs; the administrator and the medical director then have more direct responsibility for the "administrative" and "professional" activities, respectively. Regardless of organizational framework, the entire staff must be aware of the lines of responsibility.

Pediatric Service in a General Hospital

Hospitals which routinely admit infants and children should have a special unit designed exclusively for pediatrics. Children should not be admitted to adult wards, except in emergencies. A special infant unit also is recommended. When possible, special adolescent units should be provided.

If there is no adolescent unit, children 17 years of age and younger should be considered pediatric patients. The age at which a patient might be considered an adult for admitting purposes varies. However, physical and emotional maturity are important considerations in these decisions (e.g., a 14-year-old, diabetic female, pregnant for the second time, may receive better care on a high-risk obstetric service than on the pediatric division; or a 20-year-old patient with cystic fibrosis may have the physical and emotional characteristics of a young child and might be a more appropriate candidate for the pediatric unit).

As with all inpatients, a provisional diagnosis must be stated prior to the admission of pediatric patients. This facilitates appropriate placement and permits planning for necessary nursing and other personnel or equipment required during the hospitalization.

The pediatric department in general hospitals with pediatric units should be established as a separate clinical service. If one or more pediatricians are on the hospital staff, one of them should be appointed or elected as chairman of the pediatric service, with responsibility for the care rendered to children in both inpatient and outpatient settings.

Pediatric programs which are part of large general hospitals may have difficulty in developing and implementing new policy without a senior administrative representative to act as an advocate. Overall hospital policy must be carefully scrutinized at all stages of development to ensure that special circumstances which may pertain to children and adolescents have been considered. These issues are not relevant in the children's hospital setting.

Pediatric Service in a Major Teaching Hospital

Major teaching services for children will sometimes be present in large university settings. Although they may, in fact, not be separate hospitals by state licensure, they frequently are identified as separate organizational units within a university setting, with clinical excellence. They usually have a strong community identity as an autonomous facility for children. They commonly are housed in separate buildings or defined in contiguous spaces within a building reserved for the housing of children; they contain adequate clinical facilities and services for the comprehensive provision of care; and they typically have an administrative staff which functions almost exclusively in the area of pediatrics.

Children's Hospitals

The term "children's hospital" means an institution which is organized and operated specifically for the care of children and youth; the patients usually are less than 18 years old at the time of initial admission.

Where applicable, local law provides for licensing of these institutions; they are, in fact, licensed as separate and distinct hospitals which meet required standards. Thus, a free-standing children's hospital is independently accredited by the Joint Commission on Accreditation of Hospitals or by other appropriate accrediting or certifying and regulatory organizations.

Special Problems for the Administrator

Medicolegal Considerations

Consent

Generally, the law acknowledges that minors have the same rights as competent adults to privacy and access to care. However, many minors will be deemed incapable of exercising the right to consent to treatment because they lack legal competency to do so, and a parent or guardian will have the recognized right to participate in and direct appropriate decisions. In considering the sufficiency of a minor's consent, it is essential that the hospital's attorney be consulted about the requirements under the state statutes or case law.

A minor may be deemed legally capable of giving valid consent to his or her treatment, depending on the state-established doctrines surrounding the rights of married,

"emancipated," or "mature" minors. The law and judicial doctrines testing the maturity of a minor with respect to valid
consent to medical treatment vary from state to state. Generally, these tests measure the minor's capability to com-
prehend and appreciate the nature of his or her decision and
take into account the patient's chronologic age. When the
minor is married or "emancipated," there is a judicial tendency in some jurisdictions to allow a minor capable of understanding the nature and consequences of his or her action
to give valid consent to treatment. However, careful examination of the law in each jurisdiction is necessary. Situations
arise in which a minor may consent to treatment the parent
or guardian has not agreed to.

When there is a medical emergency, whether involving a
minor or an adult, a fully informed consent is not always
possible. A medical emergency occurs when there is a threat
to life or health which necessitates immediate action. If a
surrogate or guardian is available, consent must be obtained
from this person for treatment of the patient. If no parent
or surrogate is available and reasonable efforts to reach someone have proved fruitless, consent to treatment may be
legally implied from the emergency circumstances.

Refusal of consent for treatment is a situation which varies,
depending on who is refusing. If a minor refuses consent but
the parent or guardian consents, the minor's wishes should
be respected if he or she can be considered "mature" in the
jurisdiction. If a parent or guardian refuses consent but a
minor who is capable of understanding the nature of the
decision—and therefore may be considered mature—consents,
generally treatment should be given or continued. If the
minor is not mature and the parent or guardian refuses to
consent to treatment, the hospital should consult with its
attorney to determine whether there may be liability under
the state child neglect law. Court resolution of the treatment
issue may be necessary, especially if the state has a specific
neglect statute or if there are unusual circumstances, such
as a potential conflict with first amendment freedom of religious rights.

Specific note should be taken of problems of custody and
guardianship with respect to a minor's treatment. Generally,
consent must be obtained from only one parent if they are
living together, but it is preferable to get consent from both

parents. If the parents are living apart, the parent with custody usually is the one from whom consent should be obtained. When no parent or guardian is available to consent and time is critical, the person who is taking the place of the parent generally is legally authorized to consent. Because this authorization involves a legal test requiring more than mere custody, the hospital should seek legal counsel prior to accepting this type of consent.

Statutes of Limitation/Retention of Records

A statute of limitations is the prescribed period within which an injured party must bring suit after the cause of action arises. In a medical malpractice or negligence case, the cause of action usually is not deemed to have arisen until the patient knew or should have known that the injury has occurred. Statutes of limitation vary from state to state, and may vary depending on the action. For example, treating without obtaining informed consent is generally considered a battery; this may have a shorter statute-of-limitation period than the failure to disclose adequate information, which generally is a negligent action. The hospital's attorney should be consulted concerning the particular action and state statutes.

Most states have statutes which provide that the statute-of-limitation period for an injury to a minor patient does not begin until the child reaches majority. However, a parent may bring suit on the child's behalf before that time. Because the time period involved may be extremely long, careful attention must be paid to the state laws or regulations governing the required retention of records. Some states require that records of minors be preserved for a specific time after the child has reached the state-defined age of majority. Because of the constantly changing statutes, regulations, and judicial interpretations, a hospital should consult its attorney for up-to-date information.

Child Abuse

Some states provide for courts to order necessary care when parents have refused consent under a broad interpretation of child neglect. Of course, state statutes require specific actions on the part of hospitals and physicians in suspected child abuse cases. Hospitals and health care professionals must report to the appropriate public agency any actual or suspected cases of child abuse. Statutory protection from liability for negligence is provided if the child sustains additional injuries at a later date and therefore is considered to be an abused child.

Patient Rights

A child should be allowed, to the extent of his or her capacity to understand, the same rights as an adult patient. These rights, including the right to information and to privacy, may be protected by hospital policy, or by law in some states. The American Hospital Association's statement, *A Patient's Bill of Rights*,[1] offers general guidance.

Special concerns relevant to patient rights arise in a pediatric population much more frequently than for adults. The issue of who speaks for a child in medical decision making most often involves the parents and physicians. They generally represent the patient's best interests. Nonetheless, dilemmas often arise and necessitate legal action or even government involvement, although the basis for this type of intercession may be ill-defined and inconsistent. Hospitals should vest in ethics committees a major role in helping concerned parties examine all facts and options impartially, with a view toward arriving at an appropriate decision. Other examples of special circumstances in pediatrics concern the child who requires blood transfusions but whose parents' religious beliefs prohibit this, or maintaining confidentiality for the adolescent who seeks birth control or treatment of sexually transmitted diseases. Both medical and administrative staff must be informed of the law in these instances to protect the patient's rights.

Research

When a child is proposed as a subject in a project involving research, the institutional review committee should take special care to protect the child's rights. Consideration of the vulnerability of minor subjects may include greater informational requirements and special efforts to obtain unanimous consent from parents or guardian and the child. For example, the United States Department of Health and Human Services requires special protections for children involved as subjects in any research it funds or conducts. Before research is begun, a hospital should ensure that there is sensitivity to the pediatric subject's rights and welfare.

Finances

Most children's hospitals have unique financial characteristics because they usually provide much charitable or otherwise underfunded care. This results primarily from their broad geographic referral patterns and their proportion of tertiary care services, which are higher in children's hospitals than in general community facilities. Moreover, ambulatory care services provided by children's hospitals tend to serve predominantly underfunded people in urban settings.

Children's hospitals and major pediatric hospital units are unique in their staffing characteristics. Children are not young adults; their care is provided in a different fashion from that of adults. In most children's hospitals, the number of full-time personnel per bed is 4.0 to 6.0. Moreover, there are many unique personnel classifications in children's hospitals, such as child life (play) therapists, neonatal nurse practitioners, and even schoolteachers.

The pediatrics department in a general hospital often is at a disadvantage (based largely on fiscal considerations) when competing for hospital resources. Because pediatrics tends to fall among the low-income producers for hospitals, its share of the resources from among the total funds available to clinical departments frequently is inappropriately low. Competition for resources in children's hospitals may occur between divisions, some of which have the ability to produce more revenue (such as cardiology or neonatology) compared to others which cannot (such as ambulatory care). An equitable distribution of resources from the "haves" to the "have nots" is essential to ensure availability and excellence of overall medical care for infants and children.

Educational costs should be included in financial planning for teaching hospitals whether they are independent institutions (such as children's hospitals) or part of a large general hospital with university-affiliated training programs. Rarely will third party reimbursement for patient care be adequate to offset all costs. Escalating expenses for patient care exacerbate these deficiencies. Additional funds, in the form of government or foundation grants, are needed to support resident and fellowship trainees and their faculty. However, limitations on the amount of funding available from these sources have left deficits. Charitable contributions, if not committed to capital construction or equipment, can provide an additional source of funds. This may be possible through accrual of sufficient endowed funds to produce recurrent financial resources which help support educational and research missions.

Environmental Controls and Security

Adequate programs must be established to address the possibilities of internal calamities, especially fires. Of particular importance in pediatrics is an efficient evacuation plan for neonates and infants which has been tested and found effective. In addition, large pediatric departments must be prepared to deal with the problems of external disasters involving many children.

Most important, in this regard, is the organization of an efficient triage system which would expedite the appropriate level of medical care, consistent with institutional resources. Included in this consideration would be the availability of a transport system to move patients to alternate facilities, if those of the receiving institution are inadequate or exhausted. A hospital disaster committee or team is essential to developing and monitoring systems which are to be responsive to catastrophes within or outside of the hospital. The administration should provide regular and frequent disaster planning and practice for both internal disasters and community crises.

There also is a need for a well-defined security plan to protect the patients' parents, staff, and visitors, as well as the hospital property. Beyond the usual concerns of hospital security, a pediatric program with a sizable adolescent inpatient component often poses additional, specific problems. To restrain the extreme "acting-out" behavior sometimes seen among patients or their friends (especially during visiting periods), the presence of a security officer may be required. An adult companion may be required if there is a question about the patient harming him or herself. Another selective pediatric concern is the need, on rare occasions, for security when dealing with parties involved in child abuse.

In considering safety features in design of the facility, the hospital environment should be viewed the same as a home when caring for small infants and toddlers. This includes concern for the design and quality of equipment for children.

The safety of toys available for play should not be overlooked. Caution must be exercised, especially in the immediate hospital environment of infants and young toddlers, when using disinfectants and insecticides. Complete knowledge of the toxic potential of these chemicals is essential before their use is contemplated.

Special care must be given to the removal of dangerous items, including those commonly found in the home that also are used in hospitals, e.g., straight pins, thumb tacks, and sharp-tipped paper holders. Tackless bulletin boards should be used in the patient rooms, examination and treatment rooms, and at the nurses' station. Particular care is needed in the intensive care areas because the rapid pace of events may increase the risk to the patients' safety.

The architectural design of units for children should provide ample space for isolation to reduce the spread of communicable disease.

Community Relations

A favorable community image is vital to the well-being of children's medical care facilities. There should be a well-defined community relations function geared toward involving the community at all levels in supporting the specific needs of children in local general hospitals and children's hospitals in the region.

A medical institution may be heavily invested in all aspects of health care for the community in which it is located. The institution must interact with community leaders to help identify the health needs of the community and to evolve systems of health care responsive to those needs. "Visibility" in the press frequently is useful because it may help to disseminate information to the public. Dealings with the press are best conducted through an office of public information of the hospital, which can coordinate the material to be publicized and its manner of presentation. In this way, appropriate exposure can reap maximal benefits.

Fund-raising in a major institution must be coordinated through an organized, professional hospital program to avoid conflicting interests and to develop fully all leads and resources. A particularly useful form of funding is an endowment, which can provide an ongoing resource to help support medical care and educational programs.

Visiting Policies

A liberal policy for family visiting (and with adolescent patients, for friends to visit) should be encouraged. This should include visits by younger siblings in specifically designated areas. The practice of rooming-in by a parent, especially when requested, should be fostered rather than discouraged. Indeed, the concept of family-assisted care for pediatric patients should be extended. A receptive attitude toward families of children in the hospital not only benefits the morale of the patient and family, but, in a teaching hospital, it also enhances the interaction between family and house officer—an important element in the education of pediatric residents.

Medical Staff

General Rules

The care of any child admitted to a hospital should be the primary responsibility of one physician who coordinates care, obtains needed consultations, assumes responsibility for all orders, deals with family, and coordinates the final medical decision for therapy and disposition.

Rules and regulations for consultation on pediatric patients should be adopted by the medical staff of general hospitals. If a general hospital has no pediatricians on its staff, affiliation with a pediatric service in another hospital should be developed for consultation or referral.

The surgical service of a children's unit usually will have a pediatric surgeon as its chairman; when none is available, a general surgeon with interest primarily in children's surgery may be selected. General and subspecialty surgeons should be accorded pediatric privileges based on their training and experience in pediatric procedures.

The need for a pediatric medical consultation on every child surgical patient is debatable and depends on the interest, training, and experience of the surgeon. As a general rule, unless pediatric surgical specialists are involved, it is in the best interest of infants and young children to have a pediatric medical evaluation prior to major surgery and continuing medical supervision during the postoperative period.

Quality Assurance

Quality assurance must be addressed at many different levels. In a teaching program it can be approached through patient care review conferences with residents and review of the medical records. Supervision by experienced attending faculty, committed to teaching, provides one of the more vital aspects of assuring quality of care. Beyond these internal measures, results of hospital audits in compliance with state, federal, and Joint Commission on Accreditation of Hospitals requirements for monitoring and evaluating the quality and appropriateness of care add further dimension to the process of assuring quality.

Infection Control

Protection against the spread of infection is extremely important in a children's hospital. Strong, effective infection control policies, approved and followed by the medical staff as well as other care givers, provide the additional protection sick children need. An active infection control committee should be comprised of medical, laboratory, nursing, house-keeping, and administrative representatives. The program should be responsible for establishing policy, surveillance, and implementation of recommendations. If pediatrics is part of a general hospital, the infection control program must include an individual with expertise in infectious diseases of children. Infection control measures generally reflect those of the hospital but require adaptation to reflect specific problems of pediatrics.

Reference

1. Committee on Health Care for the Disadvantaged: A Patient's Bill of Rights. Chicago: American Hospital Association, 1975.

Bibliography

Statements of policy for the care of children and families in health care settings. Washington, D.C.: Association for the Care of Children in Hospitals, endorsed July 31, 1977.

Chapter 3

QUALITY ASSURANCE

Assessment of the quality of patient care and correction of identified problems have become routine functions of hospital organizations. Within recent years, political, social, and legal forces have eroded the traditional autonomy of the medical profession by mandating explicit accounting for the quality of medical care.[1] Numerous pediatricians are involved in hospital quality assurance committees in an effort to assure quality care for hospitalized children. The Academy receives inquiries about the best approach to use in evaluating the quality of care given children. The methods involved are changing, and more objective and cost-effective approaches have been developed recently.[1-4] This chapter is a review of the current state of the art of quality assurance and provides a description of useful programs available. In addition to comments on desirable qualities for quality assurance programs, references that have unique applicability to pediatric quality assurance also are given,[5-10] and commercially available resources are listed (see Addendum). Because the entire field of quality assurance still is evolving, the information in this chapter will require periodic updating.

Requirements for Quality Assurance

The goal of quality assurance is to ensure optimal patient care by monitoring, assessing, and instituting corrective action on all identified problems in patient care management. The quality assurance function currently is voluntary and reflects the ethical obligation of hospitals and the medical profession to offer the best possible care to the community. The Joint Commission on Accreditation of Hospitals (JCAH) constitutes the most prominent voluntary effort to regulate hospital quality of care. JCAH methods include setting standards, hospital surveys, and awarding of accreditation on the basis of compliance with these standards. The passage of Medicare/Medicaid legislation through enactment of the 1965

Social Security amendments established a cooperative relationship between the government and the JCAH. This legislation created "deemed status," which provided that JCAH-accredited hospitals were considered to be in compliance with conditions of participation in Medicare/Medicaid.[11]

Until 1980, the JCAH emphasis was on quality assurance review mechanisms. In 1972 the JCAH created the Performance Evaluation Procedure for Auditing and Improving Patient Care (PEP),[12] a highly organized method to assist hospitals in initiating objective quality assurance programs. Shortly after the PEP system was introduced, specific numbers of yearly audits were required. This technique proved to be a rather time-consuming paper exercise, and all too often the primary motivation of hospitals was to meet assigned quotas. Since 1977, the JCAH has been revising its quality assurance standards to encourage flexibility and innovation. Emphasis has shifted from methods to results. The 1985 standards have encouraged continuous monitoring rather than random studies.

The JCAH recognizes that many valid and useful means of review and evaluation exist and allows hospitals to select methods most pertinent and applicable to their individual situations.[11,13] The quality assurance section in the 1985 JCAH *Accreditation Manual for Hospitals*[13] defines necessary elements of quality assurance programs; therefore, it assumes remarkable significance in its effect on quality assurance and, in turn, on the care of hospitalized patients. The JCAH also publishes guidelines and resource materials.[3,14,15] Although the JCAH maintains that quality assurance programs do not need to be elaborate or expensive, a high percentage of hospitals were cited in 1982 for quality assurance deficiencies.[16]

Guidelines to the JCAH standards are well-outlined in the publication, *Back to Basics. An Introduction to Principles of Quality Assurance.*[3] A pertinent section of this book follows.

GENERAL PROVISIONS

- The governing body is responsible for the quality of care in the hospital.

- The governing body delegates responsibility to the professional and administrative staff for establishing a hospital-wide quality assurance program and assuring its effectiveness.

- This program is guided by a written plan which describes the objectives, structures, and operation of the quality assurance program.

- The scope of the quality assurance program covers all areas of direct patient care.

- Clinically valid criteria are used in the evaluation of patient care.

- Avoid duplication of effort and assure adequate attention to problems which affect more than one area of the hospital; mechanisms are in place to assure appropriate communication across departments and services and adequate follow-through on identified problems.

- The QA program oversees the effectiveness of individual quality review mechanisms.

- The structure and effectiveness of the program are evaluated and adjusted at least annually.

SPECIFIC REVIEW REQUIREMENTS

- The quality review activities outlined below should be included in a hospital's quality assurance program.

A. *Review of Credentials and Granting of Privileges*

- The medical staff periodically must review the credentials and recommend the granting of privileges for each medical staff member. This should involve an evaluation of the current competence of each practitioner and recommendations as to which procedures he/she can perform in the hospital.

B. The medical staff must establish continuous monitors of relevant aspects of their practice including:

- *Ongoing Antibiotic Review*—to examine the appropriateness of the prophylactic and therapeutic use of antibiotics

- *Monthly Surgical Case Review*—to examine the appropriateness of surgical procedures and discrepant cases

- *Quarterly Medical Record Review*—to examine the timely completion, clinical pertinence and adequacy of content of the medical record

- *Quarterly Pharmacy and Therapeutics Review*—to review and maintain drug formularies, review drug utilization, investigate drug reactions, and establish policies and procedures for the distribution and handling of drugs

- *Quarterly Blood Utilization Review*—to examine the appropriateness of the use of blood and blood products and transfusion reactions

- *Monthly Review of Care by Medical Staff Departments*—to review the care and treatment of patients including such areas as morbidity, mortality, infections and other treatment complications, and unusual or interesting cases

- *Enforcement of the Rules and Regulations of the Medical Staff*—to assure that medical staff members are abiding by the policies of their own organization

C. Hospital-Wide Functions of:

- *Infection Control*—to identify and evaluate nosocomial infections and establish and monitor aseptic and sanitation practices

- *Utilization Review*—to examine the appropriateness of admission, length of stay and identify any utilization-related problems in diagnoses, procedures, or practitioners

- *Preventive Maintenance*—to assure the safety and reliable performance of all equipment relating directly or indirectly to patient care

D. *Review and evaluation of the quality and appropriateness of nursing care*

E. *Review and evaluation of the quality and appropriateness of patient care* rendered by the following clinical support services:

- Anesthesia Services, Dietetic Services, Emergency Services, Home Care Services, Hospital-Sponsored Ambulatory Care Services, Nuclear Medicine Services, Nursing Services, Pathology and Medical Laboratory Services, Radiology Services, Rehabilitation Services, Respiratory Care, Social Work Services and Special Care Units.

The QA standard was not introduced to add some new quality assurance activity to the existing cadre of quality protective functions mentioned above but rather to encourage an organized approach, e.g., program, to review care throughout the hospital and medical staff and to provide an oversight mechanism to assure that individual functions are conducted rigorously and effectively. Three key features are critical to the success of a hospital-wide quality assurance program.

Comprehensiveness

All departments, services, committees, functions, and providers involved in the provision of care to patients participate in quality assurance activities.

Integration or Coordination of Quality Assurance Activities

Relevant information generated from QA activities is shared with appropriate hospital and medical staff, departments, committees and administration so that action can be taken at the right level to solve identified problems.

A Problem-Focused Approach

In the conduct of individual QA activities, approaches that identify, examine, and resolve problems are used. Four fundamental components characterize this process.

- Examination of key indicators or aspects of quality care

- Verification or assessment of suspected problems or concerns in care delivery to determine their cause, how pervasive they are and which departments are involved

• Implementation of corrective action

• Monitoring of follow-up to determine the effectiveness of actions taken

These standards represent an excellent list of basic qualities appropriate for any quality assurance program when combined with cost effectiveness.

Other national organizations, such as the American Hospital Association,[17,18] American Medical Association,[5] American College of Surgeons,[19,20] and Commission on Professional and Hospital Activities,[7] provide publications for use in quality assurance and utilization review programs. An example of a specialty organization which has published extensive background information and sample evaluation criteria is the American College of Obstetrics and Gynecology.[21]

Hospital quality assurance departments vary widely; the complexity commonly increases in proportion to the size of the hospital.[4] Patient record screening and other data retrieval usually are done by trained nurses or medical records technicians using objective screening criteria. However, identified variations from these criteria must still be assessed by peers. This assessment is usually performed by clinical departments or committees utilizing the services of a departmental quality assurance liaison.[2] The hospital governing body still bears the ultimate responsibility for quality of care.

Measurements of the Quality of Patient Care

Three principal measurements of the quality of patient care have traditionally been described. Many quality assessment methods include all three of these basic measurements, although some methods emphasize primarily one component.

1. Process measurement—an assessment of the procedures performed or what was done to and for the patient.

2. Outcome measurement—an assessment of the health status of the patient following medical intervention.

3. Structure measurement—an assessment of the facilities and equipment used in the care of the patient.

Process evaluation involves the setting of explicit criteria which relate to the processes of care as opposed to the outcomes. These criteria usually have a 100% standard and measure the degree to which patient management conforms to the criteria. Process criteria are based on standards and expectations of the respective health professions and accrediting bodies. Because identification of compliance with the criteria depends almost solely on documentation in the medical record, several important items (e.g., empathy, communication, and clinical judgment) may be difficult to evaluate.[1] Also, correlation of standardized processes with good outcomes has not been clearly documented.

Outcome evaluation focuses on what happened to the patient, presumably as a result of the care received. Among such outcomes are cure, normal functioning, disability, discomfort, dissatisfaction, death, or any other end result referring to some measurable aspect of health status. A system of classifying the severity of health problems has been devised to expedite measurement of change in status.[22,23] Likewise, systematic comprehensive classifications of outcome have been devised.[1,24-27] However, outcome is not totally dependent on medical intervention because many nonmedical factors are influential.

The quality of care may be influenced by the setting in which the care takes place.[10] Structure evaluation may include (1) layout and physical facilities, (2) number and category of medical personnel, and (3) safety and quality of medical devices and systems. Although certain basic facilities, staff, and equipment are necessary to deliver quality care, their presence is no guarantee of quality.

Although each of these assessment methods gives some indication of the quality of medical care, dangers and fallacies are involved in relying on a single approach to measure overall quality. Clear evidence of a cause-and-effect relationship is commonly difficult to demonstrate in each of the quality measures. A combination of methods has been suggested as the best approach to assessing medical practice, especially when applied simultaneously to all levels of hospital staff.[2,10,19,28]

Methods of Quality Assessment

Retrospective, Concurrent, and Prospective Studies

A quality of care study may be designed using retrospective, concurrent, or prospective data collection, either singly or in combination. Previously, most quality assurance studies focused on a single disease state and required retrospective chart review after the patient was discharged. A large and ever-increasing number of hospitals are adopting concurrent review systems, beginning record review shortly after admission, and continuing this review at periodic intervals while the patient is still hospitalized. Concurrent reviews' most important aspect is the ability to identify adverse patient occurrences in a timely fashion, which allows immediate corrective intervention for the patient and prevention of the same or similar adverse events in other patients.[2,19,20,29] In addition, immediate identification of and response to serious problems with potential liability is invaluable in preventing malpractice claims and subsequent losses.[30,31] Prospective audit procedures attempt to identify problems before they occur. An example is the computerized screen of all drug orders so certain errors can be identified before the drug is administered.[32]

Diagnosis and Procedure-oriented Studies

The JCAH PEP has been the most widely used and copied diagnosis-specific quality assessment method.[12] Designed as a retrospective patient chart audit, it utilizes primarily optimal outcome criteria, although critical management elements relating to specific complications are process oriented. A sample of records of patients with a specific medical diagnosis or surgical procedure is screened after discharge to identify variations. These variations are then reviewed by peers to determine whether a deficiency in care was demonstrated or whether the variations were justified. Utilization aspects are covered by criteria justifying admission, procedures, and length of stay. Other elements include complications and discharge status.

A number of systems based on the PEP retrospective diagnosis and procedure system have been developed by others (see Addendum). Some of these systems allow hospitals to combine data to develop group norms for purposes of comparison of performance in various areas.[7,33] A major problem with the retrospective diagnosis and procedure audits was the length of time required to solve problems. Examined charts were often 1 and 2 years old, and serious problems either had been continuing or were solved before the audit was done. In addition, hospitals wishing merely to meet JCAH requirements frequently selected common diagnoses and procedures in which few problems existed. The tendency for peers to justify most of the variations rather than designate deficiencies made it difficult to track more subtle problems recurring over a period of time.

Occurrence Screening Criteria Systems

In the 1970's, the proliferation of different quality assurance systems became chaotic, with a wide variety of goals, sophistication, characteristics, complexity, practicality, and cost. In some hospitals, several systems operated simultaneously in different parts of the hospital to satisfy the demands of various sponsors. Many systems were rigid and commonly required excessive physician, administrative, and personnel time. Furthermore, most systems reviewed only a small percentage of the hospital's total annual admissions and only a few diagnoses or procedures.

Simultaneously, a growing number of hospitals and physicians became self-insured, thus providing added incentive to avoid economic losses by solving medical care problems rather than allowing them to continue at their own expense. Better ways were sought to structure and utilize quality assurance methods, especially in relation to risk management. The identification of significant adverse patient occurrences became a high priority, with the objective that timely intervention could benefit the patient, the hospital, or both.[30,31,34-36]

In 1976 the California Medical Association and California Hospital Association sponsored the California Medical Insurance Feasibility Study (CMIFS) to determine the types and severity of adverse events that occur in hospitals.[37] The study showed that nearly 1 in 20 hospitalized patients experienced an adverse event that was "potentially compensable" under a no-fault system. Approximately 1% of patients admitted had an adverse occurrence which was determined to be the result of medical mismanagement. A considerable difference was noted in the data obtained by the CMIFS and data compiled by traditional diagnosis and procedure-oriented audits. The 20 general outcome screening criteria used in the CMIFS were applicable to all patient records, regardless of diagnosis, and detected adverse events frequently missed by other quality assessments based on limited numbers of diagnoses or procedures.

Increasingly, hospitals are turning to this review system, which avoids the unevenness and untimeliness of retrospective, disease and procedure-oriented audits. In this approach, a set of occurrence criteria is used to screen all patient records while patients are still in the hospital. These criteria, adapted and modified from the generic criteria used for the CMIFS, will identify 80 to 85% of all adverse patient occurrences that happen regularly in a hospital.[2,17,18,20,29,32] In addition, they may incorporate utilization review[38] and screening for all monitors required by the JCAH, e.g., tissues, transfusions, antibiotics, medical records, and hospital departmental review. Because screening is performed concurrently, peer assessments are done promptly, corrective action is more timely, and prevention of adverse occurrences has been demonstrated.[2,34,36]

Departmental and Other Miscellaneous Studies

The scope of quality assessments that could be done is large; but, in the new era of cost-containment, the effectiveness and efficiency of any system should be carefully examined. Quality assurance studies may focus on limited areas of hospital care using any of the methods outlined here. For example, drug utilization review[32,39] may include adverse drug reactions, appropriateness of drug selection, route of administration, dosage, and patient monitoring. Computers may simplify the screening of drug orders.[40] The general use of quality assurance protocols in ambulatory care has been reviewed,[41] and the special difficulties in evaluation have been noted,[1,10,42,43] especially in regard to widespread variations in the recording of data by practitioners.

Examples of other systems include department interviews and surveys, on-site personalized monitoring of a variety of patient care functions and facility adequacy,[10] clinical problem-solving algorithms,[1,41] and post-visit patient interviews and analysis of individual practitioner performance statistics.[1,43] Long-term outcome studies likewise could be accomplished. Morehead reported extensive use of expert physician reviewers who examined the entire medical record and took into account all disease and patient-related factors that bear on management decisions and results of care.[44,45] These are examples of quality assurance functions that have not enjoyed wide use, largely because of their difficulty and expense.

Patient Care Evaluation Systems

Quality assurance must be more than the application of methods for detecting substandard patient care. If assessment and action do not logically follow detection, quality assurance becomes a mere paper exercise. Increasing emphasis is now being placed on systems which incorporate all essential elements. In the systems approach, all quality assurance-related activities are integrated into a hospitalwide organization with a single point of accountability. Among the activities which should be integrated are utilization review,[38,46] continuing medical education,[4,19,49] risk management,[31,47,48] infection control, hospital department functions (e.g., nursing, pharmacy,[32,39] medical records, public relations[19]), and medical staff functions such as reappointment and delineation of clinical privileges, monitoring of antibiotic/drug utilization, and transfusion and tissue review.

A good occurrence screening system supplemented with internal reporting mechanisms, e.g., incident reports, transmittals, and other data sources, can provide adequate information for all of these areas. This opens channels of communication between various medical staff committees and hospital departments to solve problems through coordinated action. Although each clinical discipline has responsibility for identifying and solving problems related to patient care in its area, many problems are multidisciplinary, and coordination of the overall quality assurance program is often best performed by a single committee, group, or individual. Setting priorities and collection of all quality assurance-related data by a centralized quality assurance/utilization review/risk management department will eliminate overlapping reviews by different hospital services. Expeditious peer review of all adverse events should be included in the system, as well as a strong organizational structure to deal with identified problems. A number of systems are now being described in the literature.[2,19,29,30,36]

Relationship Between Quality Assurance and Improvement in Patient Care

Continued improvement of quality of care attributed directly to traditional quality assurance activities has not been definitively demonstrated.[1,49] For example, proving that all the recommended diagnostic and therapeutic procedures in any given diagnosis-oriented medical audit relate to a better outcome for the patient is difficult. Hence, criteria may lack validity.[10,42,43] Guidelines for setting valid criteria exist but are seldom used, and some studies show that correlations between processes and clinical outcomes are generally weak.[1] However, properly designed evaluations can demonstrate strong statistical associations between validated procedures and clinical outcomes.[49] Recent studies show dramatic improvement in physician behavior and patient outcomes when comprehensive, objective practice review is combined with individual practitioner counseling.[50]

In theory, each review should provide feedback regarding quality of care, and the responsible persons in the organization should assure that problems are solved.[16] Otherwise, the data collection is of little value. Serious adverse patient occurrences may be isolated or part of an evolving pattern of substandard care; they may involve a single practitioner or employee, or they may be multidisciplinary and systemwide. An effective quality assurance program can classify all these events for appropriate action so the hospital and medical staff can demonstrate accountability.

Legal Issues

Several court cases have established the precedent that hospital organizations are responsible for the quality of care of their patients. Most states have enacted laws designed to protect committee members engaging in quality assurance activities from legal liability (with certain qualifications) and to limit discovery or admissibility of the work of the committee.[31] However, these laws vary in content from state to state.[51]

The statements of medical staff members involved are protected at common law by a "qualified privilege." Communications must be made in good faith, without malice and with reasonable care to ascertain the truth of the matter. All information should be reported accurately and fairly, and only to persons with legitimate interest.[18]

Medical staff applicants and members should be required to release committee members and other hospital personnel from civil liability for alleged harm arising from the discharge of official evaluation duties. Whenever quality assurance findings are used in processing medical staff applications for appointment and reappointment, initiating corrective action, and pursuing due process elements, faithful adherence to hospital bylaws is necessary. Hospitals commonly carry insurance to protect committee members against potential liability arising from such services as quality assurance activities.[18]

Conclusions and Recommendations

Hospital quality assurance is an activity worthy of widespread involvement by pediatricians. The advent of prospective payment mechanisms in hospital patient care may provide increased impetus for effective quality assurance; however, the most important motivation should continue to be the physician's ethical desire to prevent injury and promote quality for patients. Appropriate quality assurance mechanisms may help protect the physician from potential abuse from prospective pricing programs. Areas of abuse might include undue pressure for early patient discharge and selection of medical staff on the basis of economics. The JCAH emphasis on hospitalwide integration, problem-focused studies, continuous monitoring, and follow-up action has stimulated the development of more efficient systems for carrying out these responsibilities in recent years. Because of this rapid development of quality assurance methods and the ready availability of effective resources, the Academy no longer publishes sample criteria sets. Quality assurance program characteristics necessary for hospital accreditation are explicitly defined by the JCAH. A number of choices are available for systems which fulfill all requirements. A promising development in quality assurance is occurrence screening of patient records using standardized criteria applicable to concurrent or retrospective review of all patient admissions. These occurrence screening criteria have been modified to apply to all services, including pediatrics. Quality assurance resources may be used more efficiently by screening records for all aspects of patient care, utilization, and risk management simultaneously rather than performing these required activities in a fragmented, time-consuming manner. Pediatricians and hospital departments need only review important, identified problems and trends and thus have more time available for effective action. Flexibility must be maintained in the quality assurance arena as new concepts are developed to assess health care provided to children in hospitals.

Addendum

Useful Resources for Hospital Quality Assurance Programs*

General Overview of Quality Assurance and Technical Information

American College of Surgeons: Patient Safety Manual. Chicago: American College of Surgeons, 1979.

Donabedian, A.: The Definition of Quality and Approaches to Its Assessment (Explorations in Quality Assessment and Monitoring Series). Ann Arbor, Michigan: Health Administration Press, 1980.

Orlikoff, J.E., Fifer, W.R., and Greeley, H.P.: Malpractice Prevention and Liability Control for Hospitals. Chicago: American Hospital Association, 1981.

Skillicorn, S.A.: Quality and Accountability: A New Era in American Hospitals. San Francisco: Editorial Consultants, Inc., 1980.

Williams, K.J., and Donnelly, P.R. Medical Care Quality and the Public Trust (Teach 'em), Chicago: Pluribus Press, 1982.

Gonnella, J.S., ed.: Clinical Criteria for Disease Staging. Santa Barbara, California: SysteMetrics, 1983.

Graham, N.O., ed.: Quality Assurance in Hospitals: Strategies for Assessment and Implementation. Rockville, Maryland: Aspen, 1982.

Diagnosis and Procedure Medical Audits

The CHAMP Comparative Pediatric Audit System. Alexandria, Virginia: Children's Hospitals Automated Medical Programs (CHAMP) (c/o NACHRI, 325 First Street), 1984.

Audit Criteria Series, Issue No. 1-8, Chicago: InterQual. (Various issues in the series contain audit criteria for pediatrics, OB/Gyn, anesthesia, mastectomy, transfusion, and many other procedures. Dates of publication vary.)

---

*This list is not necessarily all-inclusive of available programs. This listing does not imply endorsement by the American Academy of Pediatrics. Please note dates of publications as some criteria will need updating. Even though some programs are out of print, they are commonly available in hospital libraries or quality assurance offices.

Sample Criteria for Procedure Review: Screening Criteria to Assist PSROs. Baltimore: Department of Health and Human Services, 1981.
Reference Criteria for Short-Stay Hospital Review. Baltimore: Department of Health and Human Services, 1980.

Occurrence Screening Criteria Systems

Craddick, J.W.: Medical Management Analysis: A Systematic Approach to Quality Assurance and Risk Management, Volume I: An Introduction, 1983, and Volume II: An Implementation Manual, 1984. Auburn, California: Joyce W. Craddick, M.D. (Department 10, 24654 Rodeo Flat Road).
Identifying and Analyzing Clinically Related Occurrences. Chicago: InterQual, Inc., 1982.
American College of Surgeons (in consultation with Maryland Hospital Education Institute): Providing Management Information for Patient Safety Programs. Chicago: American College of Surgeons, 1980.
American Hospital Association: QTM-80 Programs. Chicago: American Hospital Association, 1980.
The Masters Manual. Chicago: Care Communications Inc. (233 East Erie Street).
Hospital Risk Management and Malpractice Liability Control. Chicago: InterQual, Inc., 1980.

Helpful Periodicals

Quality Review Bulletin (QRB—the journal of quality assurance). JCAH, 875 N. Michigan Avenue, Chicago, Illinois 60611.
Hospital Peer Review. American Health Consultants, Inc., 67 Peachtree Park Drive, N.E., Atlanta, Georgia 30309.
Medical Management Analysis Information Digest. Joyce W. Craddick, M.D., Department 10, 24654 Rodeo Flat Road, Auburn, California 95603.
QA/RM Bulletin. Maryland Hospital Education Institute, 1309 York Road, Lutherville, Maryland 21093.
Quality Assurance Plan: Hospital Pediatrics Department, Medical Newsletter and Update Service, Inc., P.O. Box 8, 202 East Main, Marion, Illinois 62959.

References

1. Sanazaro, P.J.: Quality assessment and quality assurance in medical care. Ann. Rev. Pub. Health, 1:37, 1980.
2. Craddick, J.W.: Medical Management Analysis: A Systematic Approach to Quality Assurance and Risk Management. Volume I: An Introduction. Auburn, California: Joyce W. Craddick, M.D., 1983.
3. Mikolzjczak, A., Nagel, L.J., and Walczak, R.: Back to Basics. An Introduction to Principles of Quality Assurance. Chicago: Joint Commission on Accreditation of Hospitals, 1982.
4. Shanahan, M.: Patient care evaluation: Coming of age in the 80's. QRB, 7:10, April 1981.
5. American Medical Association: Sample Criteria for Procedure Review: Screening Criteria to Assist PSROs. Chicago: American Medical Association, 1981.
6. Bass, J.L., Mehta, K.A., Gordon, M.J., et al.: A pediatric ambulatory care evaluation. QRB, 7:9, August 1981.
7. Commission on Professional and Hospital Activities: Length of Stay by Diagnosis, by Operation, Pediatrics 1982. Ann Arbor, Michigan: Commission on Professional and Hospital Activities, 1984.
8. Hurwitz, L.S., and Kohler, E.: The benefits of evaluating care provided to children hospitalized with insulin dependent diabetes mellitus. QRB, 7:13, June 1981.
9. Craddick, J.W., ed: Medical Management Analysis Information Digest, Pediatric Edition, Volume II, No. 2. Auburn, California: Joyce W. Craddick, M.D., March 1984.
10. Osborne, C.E., and Thompson, H.C.: Criteria for evaluation of ambulatory child health care by chart audit: Development and testing of a methodology. Final report of the Joint Committee on Quality Assurance of Ambulatory Health Care for Children and Youth. Pediatrics, 56:625, 1975.
11. Affeldt, J.E.: Struggle for the assurance of appropriate medical care. Bull. N.Y. Acad. Med., 58:39, January-February, 1982.
12. P.E.P. Primer, ed. 2. Chicago: Joint Commission on Accreditation of Hospitals, 1975.
13. Joint Commission on Accreditation of Hospitals: Accreditation Manual for Hospitals, 1985. Chicago: Joint Commission on Accreditation of Hospitals, 1984.
14. Making QA Work for You! Chicago: Joint Commission on Accreditation of Hospitals, revised 1982.
15. The QA Guide. A Resource for Hospital Quality Assurance. Chicago: Joint Commission on Accreditation of Hospitals, 1980.

16. Children's Hospitals Automated Medical Programs: Health care trends: CHAMP Update. Hosp. Peer Rev., 8:45, December 1982.
17. American Hospital Association: QTM-81 Programs. Chicago: American Hospital Association, 1981.
18. American Hospital Association: The Quality Assurance Program for Medical Care in the Hospital (QAP). Chicago: American Hospital Association, 1972.
19. American College of Surgeons (in consultation with Maryland Hospital Education Institute): American College of Surgeons Patient Safety Manual. Chicago: American College of Surgeons, 1979.
20. American College of Surgeons (in consultation with Maryland Hospital Education Institute): Providing Management Information for Patient Safety Programs. Chicago: American College of Surgeons, 1980.
21. American College of Obstetrics and Gynecology: Quality Assurance in Obstetrics and Gynecology. Chicago: American College of Obstetrics and Gynecology, 1980.
22. Gonella, J.S., and Goran, M.J.: Quality of patient care—A measurement of change: The staging concept. Med. Care, 13:467, 1975.
23. Gonella, J.S., ed.: Clinical Criteria for Disease Staging. Santa Barbara, California: SysteMetrics, Inc., 1983.
24. Brook, R.H., Davies-Avery, A., Greenfield, S., et al.: Assessing the quality of medical care using outcome measures: An overview of the method. Med. Care, 15:1, 1977.
25. Howe, M.J., Coulton, M.R., and Almon, G.M.: Use of scaled outcome criteria for a target patient population. QRB, 6:15, 20, April 1980.
26. Sanazaro, P.J., and Williamson, J.W.: End results of patient care: A provisional classification based on reports by internists. Med. Care, 6:123, 1968.
27. Sanazaro, P.J., ed.: Private Initiative in Professional Standards Review Organizations (PSRO): Final Report. Ann Arbor, Michigan: Health Administration Press, 1978.
28. Skillicorn, S.A.: Quality and Accountability: A New Era in American Hospitals. San Francisco: Editorial Consultants, Inc., 1980.
29. Craddick, J.W.: Medical Management Analysis: A Systematic Approach to Quality Assurance and Risk Management. Volume II: An Implementation Manual. Auburn, California: Joyce W. Craddick, M.D., 1984.
30. Craddick, J.W.: The medical management analysis system: A professional liability warning mechanism. QRB, 5:2, April 1979.

31. Craddick, J.W.: Use existing motivations to involve physicians in risk management. Hospitals, 55:63, 85, June 1, 1981.
32. Stolar, M.H.: The case for prospective and concurrent drug utilization review. QRB, 8:6, June 1982.
33. Macaluso, D., Stein, B., and Polster, L.R.: CHAMP: A comparative study approach. QRB, 6:19, July 1980.
34. Jones, D., and Bader, K.: Innovative QA program improves care and decreases cost. Hosp. Peer Rev., 6:73, July 1981.
35. McCollum, W.E.: Multifacility program addresses both QA and risk management. Hospitals, 55:96, June 1, 1981.
36. White, J.S.: Is this the ultimate step in quality control? Med. Econom., 60:204, 1983.
37. California Medical Association and California Hospital Association: Report on the Medical Insurance Feasibility Study. San Francisco: Sutter Publications, Inc., 1977.
38. The ISDA Review System. Chicago: InterQual, Inc., 1984.
39. Christopherson, R.C., and Grant, K.L.: Drug Utilization Monitoring and Educational Parameters. Madison, Wisconsin: University of Wisconsin Hospitals and Clinics, Department of Pharmacy, 1981.
40. Stolar, M.H.: National survey of hospital pharmaceutical services—1978. Amer. J. Hosp. Pharm., 36:316, 1979.
41. Komaroff, A.L., Ervin, C.T., Pass, T.M., and Sherman, H.: Protocols in ambulatory care. Pub. Health Rev., 7:135, 1978.
42. Hill, R.K.: Quality assurance in ambulatory care. Primary Care, 7:713, 1980.
43. Palmer, R.H., and Nesson, H.R.: A review of methods for ambulatory medical care evaluations. Med. Care, 20:758, 1982.
44. Morehead, M.A., and Donaldson, R.: Quality of clinical management of disease in comprehensive neighborhood health centers. Med. Care, 12:301, 1974.
45. Morehead, M.A.: The medical audit as an operational tool. Amer. J. Pub. Health, 57:1643, 1967.
46. Sandrick, K.M.: Private review—Its impact on health care and physicians. QRB, 8:5, April 1982.
47. Collins, P.: Hospital aims quality assurance, risk management education at staff. Hospitals, 55:93, June 1, 1981.
48. Orlikoff, J.E., and Lanham, G.B.: Why risk management and quality assurance should be integrated. Hospitals, 55:54, June 1, 1981.
49. Sanazaro, P.J., and Worth, R.M.: Concurrent quality assurance in hospital care: Report of a study by private initiative in PSRO. New Engl. J. Med., 298:1171, 1978.

50. Craddick, J.W.: Demonstrated Improvement in Physician Behavior and Patient Management Utilizing Objective Chart Review and Constructive Counseling. Unpublished manuscript.
51. Chennen, A.: Hospitals have legal duty to assure quality of health care. Hosp. Peer Rev., 7:148, December 1982.

Chapter 4

DELINEATION OF PRIVILEGES IN
HOSPITALS*

In 1973 the Committee on Hospital Care published a statement entitled, "Delineation of Pediatric Privileges in Hospitals."[1] Since then there have been many new developments
in this area, and there is increasing litigation.[2] Many pediatricians are involved not only as individual physicians but
also as members of, or advisors to, hospital departmental
committees, medical staffs, and hospital governing bodies in
decisions about the general delineation of privileges, specific
medical staff appointments, and granting of privileges. Every
pediatrician practicing hospital medicine is subject to this
process. In view of the continued evolution and increasing
importance of this field, the following review and guidelines
are offered.

The evolving legal doctrines of hospital corporate liability
generally provide that a hospital governing body is responsible for the maintenance of proper standards of professional
work in the hospital and for the functioning of the medical
staff in conformity with reasonable standards of competency.[3,4] The hospital credentialing process is one method by
which hospital governing bodies meet their legal responsibilities and strive to protect patients from incompetent or
unqualified physicians.[2,3,5] The hospital governing body has
overall responsibility for the quality of patient care,[6] but it
delegates to the medical staff the duty to recommend only
competent physicians to treat patients in the hospital.[3,6-8] A
physician does not have the right to practice in any hospital
he or she chooses; rather, each hospital grants permission or
the privilege to practice therein.[2,3,9] The Joint Commission
on Accreditation of Hospitals (JCAH) considers credentialing

*Adapted from: Committee on Hospital Care: Delineation of Pediatric
Privileges in Hospitals, Pediatrics, 70:813, 1982.

to be a major hospital quality assurance measure and an important factor in hospital risk management.[10]

Initial Appointment

When a physician joins a hospital medical staff, two processes are usually involved: initial appointment and the granting of initial clinical privileges. The former is the granting of a request from a physician to become a member of the organized medical staff under one or more of several possible categories. The criteria for appointment involve data that indicate the candidate generally should be able to perform competently as a staff physician.[6,7]

Clinical Privileges

A related but distinct process involves the defining and granting of specific pediatric privileges. Becoming a member of a medical staff does not denote the right of an individual to practice the entire spectrum of medicine and surgery in that hospital. To the contrary, the right to perform individual procedures or provide specific types of care must be requested by the prospective member, and it is the responsibility of the hospital medical staff and hospital governing board to assure that the physician meets a reasonable standard of competency in the requested areas of practice.[6] Privileges should be granted on the basis of training, experience, judgment, and demonstrated clinical competence.[6,11]

Recommendations for pediatric privileges commonly emanate from a pediatric departmental committee. It is necessary to have independent review of the recommendations by multidisciplinary, impartial, and influential groups such as the medical staff executive and credentials committees. The procedure for appointment to the medical staff and granting of pediatric privileges must be defined in the medical bylaws, rules, and regulations; and it must be followed carefully. Final approval of actions in both areas lies with the governing body.[6,12]

Documentation of Competence

The JCAH guidelines state:

Unless otherwise provided by law, only those physicians and dentists holding an appropriate license and offering evidence ... adequate to assure the medical staff and governing body that any patient treated by them will receive optimal achievable quality of care (should) be eligible for medical staff membership.

Evidence must reflect demonstrated current clinical competence and must be verified. Minimum documentation must include information relative to medical school and postgraduate training, professional experience, references from persons knowledgeable about the applicant's competence and ethical character, and current licensure. The JCAH strongly recommends documentation of adverse malpractice action, challenges to licensure or registration, loss of medical organization membership, and loss of medical staff membership or privileges at another hospital.[6] A statement regarding the nature of previous privileges in other hospitals,[7] physical and mental health, and documentation of specialty board certification may be requested as well.[3,6,12]

Causes for concern include high mobility, graduation from certain foreign medical schools, malpractice suits, and professional disciplinary actions. In some instances there may be need for extensive written documentation and verification by telephone or other means.[7] Documents can be falsified, and vital information purposefully omitted by applicants. Inquiry into court records for malpractice information may be necessary.[2]

The granting of appropriate privileges demands careful documentation that the applicant has the specific training and experience to perform the procedures and treat the diseases requested. Care should be taken in areas in which proficiency and safety are attained only by continuing experience. When delineation of privileges is based primarily on experience, adequate documentation of specific experience and successful results should be obtained.[6]

Monitoring

Monitoring each staff member during the period of provisional staff membership and monitoring members requesting additional privileges add credibility to the credentialing process. When evaluating competency, there is no substitute for direct observation of clinical skills. Recommendations include: the policy for monitoring should be defined in the bylaws, rules, and regulations (each department may wish to establish its own monitoring protocols); monitoring should apply to all new staff members; direct observation is preferable to chart review; a minimum duration or number of cases should be specified; a sufficient number and variety of cases should be observed to demonstrate necessary skills, depending on the scope of clinical privileges requested; the physician monitors should submit written evaluations; more than one person should act as monitor; monitoring should include all aspects of patient management, including chart review, direct observation of invasive procedures, and observation of diagnostic and treatment techniques; and the physician monitors should have sufficient expertise to evaluate the quality of care provided.[13]

Use of Criteria

The methods for granting or restricting of medical privileges should be reasonable and noncapricious, and should avoid reliance on subjective impressions. Irrelevant, arbitrary, or inconsistent criteria should be avoided, and the criteria which are used should not be applied inconsistently to different individuals. Criteria based on sex, race, creed, or national origin;[6] membership in certain professional societies; or membership in a prepaid, closed-panel group practice should be avoided.[7] Courts have decided in favor of physicians who have sued hospitals when their appointments or clinical privileges have been denied on the basis of such inappropriate criteria.[1,14]

Privileges should not depend on any single criterion such as Board certification or membership in a specialty society.[3,5,15] Physicians from various specialties may rightfully be allowed to treat the same diseases and perform the same procedures if they meet appropriate criteria.[5,6,11,15-18] Jurisdictional disputes should be discouraged in favor of rational granting of privileges. Specialty Board qualification and certification may, however, serve as useful benchmarks in granting privileges.[6]

Criteria should relate reasonably to standards of patient care or to the objectives and purposes of the institution. Several items beyond the scope of this paper have been reviewed elsewhere: exclusive arrangements between hospitals and physicians; exclusion of physicians on the basis of unavailable bed space or overabundance of certain specialists; moral, ethical, and behavioral considerations;[14] and the relationship of privileging to antitrust laws.[19,20]

Specifying Clinical Privileges

There are several ways of specifying clinical privileges. A once-popular method was the use of broad categories such as "surgery," "medicine," or "pediatrics," without further defining a physician's activity in that area. Such broad generalization is now considered too nonspecific to define a physician's activities commensurate with his or her training and experience.[6]

A horizontal and vertical approach to privileging has been described. For example, a physician may request privileges in a number of categories such as surgery, medicine, and pediatrics (or in certain subspecialties). Within each category, classifications are developed to reflect complexity of patient care. Thus, the horizontal dimension reflects arenas of patient care activity, and the vertical dimension reflects the degree of skill involved.[21]

The list approach is the most commonly used method of defining degrees of skill. Physicians are presented a list of medical and surgical procedures and/or disease states and asked to indicate those in which they feel qualified. Although specific, the list approach may be exhaustive and difficult to manage. It is especially difficult for the surgical specialties to produce lists that are all-inclusive.[22] The lists should be long enough to define clearly the scope of a practitioner's activities, but they should not be so detailed as to result in hairsplitting.[6,21]

Another method of defining degrees of skill is termed the level approach. It refines the list approach by outlining groups or levels of procedures or diseases based on progressive difficulty and complexity. For example, hematologic diseases might progress from level 1, exemplified by iron-deficiency anemia, to level 4, exemplified by monocytic leukemia. A family physician or pediatrician might qualify for level 1, and a pediatrician who is Board certified in hematology/oncology might qualify for levels 1 through 4. Other disease groups might have similar levels. Practitioners would be free to request privileges at whichever level they feel qualified within each disease grouping, and they would perform certain procedures commensurate with performance at that particular level.[7]

A variation of the level approach is to define levels or categories of physician competency rather than levels of disease. These categories may be based on special training or Board certification in specialties or subspecialties, or on equivalent experience. Appropriate levels of diseases or procedures to be handled by the practitioner are generated on the basis of level of training rather than vice versa.[16]

Physicians have been granted privileges on the basis of whether the circumstance requires supervision or consultation.[16,23] Methods that classify illnesses and/or procedures into groups allow flexibility and generalization that fixed lists do not; however, it has been suggested that a combination of the category and list approach may be the best method to delineate privileges.[3,16,17]

The JCAH allows considerable latitude in the type of method used for defining privileges.[6] There is no requirement of a complicated "laundry list," but the JCAH permits a listing of procedures or medical diseases as one possible alternative. Surveyor guidelines require evidence of "adequate documentation of previous training and experience, clinical privilege request forms that at least identify the specialty areas designated by the specialty board, and documentation indicating an effort has been made to match expertise with clinical privileges to the extent that is practical for the individual hospital in view of its location, range of services, and the availability of medical manpower." The medical staff bylaws may allow each staff member the privilege of performing emergency lifesaving procedures.

Useful and comprehensive reviews of the process for granting privileges have been published.[3,7,12]

Reissuance of Clinical Privileges

Periodic reappointment to the medical staff and review of privileges is a necessity in view of changing capabilities of practitioners (ordinarily not more than every 2 years).[6] Reissuing of privileges may be done at any time a significant change in a physician's ability to practice medicine is noted. Renewal of privileges should be recognized by the entire medical staff as a continuing and necessary function applying to all members, and as subject to the same necessity for objectivity and fairness as the initial granting of privileges.

The *Accreditation Manual for Hospitals*[6] states:

Reappointment policies shall provide for appraisal of each member of the staff at the time of reappointment. The appraisal shall include information relative to the individual's professional performance, judgment, and, when appropriate, technical skill. The appraisal shall also include consideration of the staff member's health status.

Appropriate factors for reappraisal of medical staff include continuing medical education; timely, accurate, and complete medical records; attendance at required staff and departmental meetings; service on hospital committees as requested; and patterns of care as demonstrated by hospital evaluations.[6] Exchange of information regarding physician performance between hospital departments may be helpful.

Privileges may be expanded when there is further training or clinical experience. Modification or rescinding of privileges may be indicated if the physician has repeated or significant deficiencies in particular areas identified on medical care evaluation studies, and if counseling or reeducation has not been effective. The retrospective medical audit also may provide objective criteria to allow a dispassionate appraisal of the staff member's competence.[3,15,24] It is common for practitioners to ask for modification of the requested privileges at the time of periodic review, in recognition of their own changing skills. Supervision by members of the medical staff of a number of clinical cases at the time of reissuance of privileges may be considered. Careful plans for renewal of privileges have been devised for physicians of retirement age.[24,25]

Due Process

Should a hospital organization decide to deny staff appointment or reappointment—or deny, curtail, or suspend privileges—it is imperative that due process and equal protection are provided in accordance with customary legal principles and as defined, where appropriate, in the hospital medical staff bylaws. Two types of due process exist: substantive and procedural. Substantive due process is concerned with whether the rules and criteria stipulated in the bylaws are reasonable, fair, and not arbitrary, and whether the decisions made by a hospital medical staff or hearing panel are based on the weight of relevant and reliable evidence and only on that evidence which is presented to the medical staff or hearing panel. Procedural due process is concerned with whether such rules are properly administered and applied equally to all staff members. A formal appeals process must be available to each candidate.[3,6] In view of increasing litigation in this area, consultation with an attorney may help to guarantee due process before the final action is taken.[7,14]

General Practitioners, Family Physicians, and Nonpediatricians

Granting pediatric privileges to general practitioners, family physicians, and nonpediatrician specialists may impose dilemmas. Exposure to pediatrics in the various training programs is variable. It may be helpful to request a response from the training program of a nonpediatrician applicant regarding the appropriateness of his or her set of requested privileges. Some residency programs document residents' exposure to disease entities and procedures; this may be help-ful.[26] A statement from the applicant indicating his or her qualifications to perform each item on the checklist has been suggested as a requirement.[17] For an applicant who has had practice experience, responses by physicians with knowledge of the practitioner's capabilities are useful.

Limited pediatric privileges are commonly granted to non-pediatrician physicians through emergency room, family practice, surgery, and other departmental committees. The Committee on Hospital Care suggests that these privileges should be granted by the physician's primary committee, but with the advice and consent of the pediatric committee (in departmentalized hospitals). All applicants should be subject to the same criteria and privilege-granting process, including monitoring, regardless of the sponsoring committee.

Nonphysician Health Professionals

Pressure to grant hospital clinical privileges to nonphysician health professionals is increasing. Many such professionals are being trained to provide services previously provided only by physicians. The evolving status of hospital privileges for these groups has been reviewed.[27] The responsibility of the hospital organization to allow only competent individuals to engage in hospital health care also extends to this category of practitioner.[27]

The *Accreditation Manual for Hospitals*[6] of the JCAH states:

The medical staff shall delineate in its bylaws, rules and regulations the qualifications, status, clinical duties, and responsibilities of specified professional personnel whose services require that they be processed through the usual medical staff channels. This should be performed in consultation with the chief executive officer on a categorical rather than an individual basis. The training, experience, and demonstrated current competence of individuals in such categories shall be sufficient to permit their performing the following: the exercising of judgment within their areas of competence, providing that a physician member of the medical staff shall have the ultimate responsibility for patient care; participating directly in the management of patients under the supervision or direction of a member of the medical staff, and within the limits established by the medical staff and consistent with the State Practice Acts; the writing of orders and the recording of reports and progress notes in patients' medical records.

These practitioners may include house staff, physician's assistants, nurse practitioners, nurse anesthetists, midwives, psychologists, doctoral scientists,[10] and others.

The JCAH states that membership on the medical staff, subject to applicable state law, is limited to physicians and dentists.[6] The nonphysician health professional should be accredited through the regular physician staff mechanism, with final approval of the governing body. The extent of their final roles and functions should be recommended by the medical staff. The nonphysician health professional must comply with the hospital bylaws, rules, and regulations.[6,27]

Individual nonphysician health professionals should be assigned to appropriate clinical departments and should be subject to departmental policies. It may be appropriate for the staff bylaws to provide for staff affiliate status.[12,27] Continuous monitoring of the nonphysician health professional's hospital activity should be implemented,[27] as well as a mechanism for renewal of privileges.

Summary

The initial statement and format suggested by the Committee on Hospital Care in 1973 has been used successfully in its present form or in modified form throughout the United States. It combines a list approach with a level of competence approach. This general format is still appropriate, but it constitutes only one of several alternatives available. The Addendum provides an example of current modification of the 1973 format. Most important is that the principles are followed to protect the patient, hospital, and physician through the process of delineation of hospital privileges.

References

1. Committee on Hospital Care: Delineation of pediatric privileges in hospitals. News and Comment (Suppl. 6), Vol. 24. July 1973.
2. Hospital privilege issue examined in AMA counsel's talk. AAFP Reporter, p. 8, June 1981.
3. Joint Commission on Accreditation Quality Review Center:

Defining Clinical Privileges for the Hospital Medical Staff. Chicago: JCAH, pp. 1-42, 1974 (out of print).

4. Southwick, A.F.: The legal perspectives. Trustee, 29:7, 1976.

5. American Board of Medical Specialties: ABMS Statement on Delineation of Staff Privileges. Approved by Executive Committee of ABMS, January 28, 1977.

6. Joint Commission on Accreditation of Hospitals: Accreditation Manual for Hospitals, 1982 ed. Chicago: JCAH, 1981.

7. Appointment and clinical privileges: Role and responsibilities of the Board of Trustees. Adapted from Hospital Trustee Development Program. American Hospital Association, 1979. QRB, 6:5, 1980.

8. Joint Commission on Accreditation of Hospitals: "Laundry lists" inessential to clinical privileging. Perspect. Accredit., 6:3, November-December, 1977.

9. Brosseau, H.L.: A privilege is not a right. Dimens. Health. Serv., 51:4, 1974.

10. Affeldt, J.E.: JCAH requirements for delineation of clinical privileges and duties. Hosp. Med. Staff, 9:7, 1980.

11. Jurisdictional Disputes Among Medical Specialties: AMA Resolution 88, p. 274, adopted July 22-26, 1979, 128th Annual Meeting; AMA Resolution 11, p. 215, adopted June 7-11, 1981, 130th Annual Meeting.

12. Blalock, W.R.: Delineation of privileges in a university teaching hospital. Case Stud. Health Adm., 2:145, 1980.

13. CMA Medical Staff Survey Committee: CMA Guidelines for Medical Staff Proctoring. Approved by CMA Council, August 1978, revised June 1979.

14. Southwick, A.F.: Due process. I. The physician's right to due process and equal protection. Hosp. Med. Staff, 7:30, 1978.

15. Statement on qualifications for surgical privileges in approved hospitals. Bull. Amer. Coll. Surg., 62:12, 1977.

16. Delineating hospital privileges by the medical staff. Bull. Amer. Coll. Phys., pp. 13-15, June 1975.

17. American Society of Internal Medicine: Delineation of Hospital Medical Staff Privileges. ASIM publication No. 324; approved by Board of Trustees, February 1980.

18. American Academy of Facial Plastic and Reconstructive Surgery: Delineation of Hospital Privileges for the Practice of Head and Neck Plastic Surgery, undated.

19. Pollard, M.R.: The essential role of antitrust in a competitive market for health services. Milbank Mem. Fund Q., 59:256, 1981.

20. Pollard, M.R., and Leinbenluft, R.E.: Antitrust and the Health Professions. Policy Planning, Issues Paper. Federal Trade Commission Office of Policy Planning, pp. 92-106, July 1981.

21. Felch, W.C.: Views from the chairman: The privilege's problem. Hosp. Med. Staff, 5:18, 1976.
22. Patz, S.M.: Privilege delineation system leaves room for flexibility. Hosp. Med. Staff, 9:2, 1980.
23. Girard, N.E.: Consultation requirement defines privileges, refines care. Hosp. Med. Staff, 3:10, 1974.
24. Brewer, J.I., and Porterfield, J.D.: Restriction of privileges for the aging surgeon. J.A.M.A., 230:613, 1974.
25. Pemberton, L.B.: Surgical privileges for retirement-age surgeons in a community hospital. Bull. Amer. Coll. Surg., 59:12, 1974.
26. Terrell, H.P.: Documentation of resident exposure to disease entities. J. Fam. Pract., 6:317, 1978.
27. Porter, J.T.: Hospital privileges for nonphysicians raise hard legal questions. Hosp. Med. Staff, 7:22, 1978.

Addendum

Delineation of Pediatric Privileges

Pediatric Privileges Requested by _____
    Board Qualified _____ Staff Category _____
    Board Certified _____ Department _____
    Subspecialty Board Qualified _____ or Certified _____

Please check all categories and privileges desired.

I. Pediatric privileges (privileges to perform emergency lifesaving procedures are automatically granted to all staff physicians):

____ Category 0
Privileges usually granted a nonpediatrician specialty consultant who, in the opinion of the attending physician and chief of pediatrics, is capable of performing diagnostic consultation and/or specialty services urgently needed in the care of a critically ill patient or one with a diagnostic problem.

____ Category 1
Illness or problem with no apparent serious threat to life. This category is usually granted to family physicians or internists.

____ Category 2
Illness or problem requiring skills usually acquired

after 1 year of pediatric training or its equivalent in experience.

___ Category 3

Complex or severe illness or potentially life-threatening problems usually requiring skills acquired after pediatric training sufficient for Board eligibility/certification or its equivalent in experience.

___ Category 4

Intensive care of children, including ventilatory care and advanced life support.

___ Category 5

Illness or problem requiring expertise acquired only during subspecialty training or similar experience. Subspecialty practice: _____

(This category does not necessarily include all others. Please check other categories desired.)

II. Neonatal care privileges:

___ Class A

(For those requesting Category 1, 2, 3 or 4) Normal care of newborn infants >2,000 gm.

___ Class B

(For those requesting Category 3 or 4) Care of preterm or low-birth-weight infants with nonlife-threatening illness, and not requiring ventilatory support.

___ Class C

(For those requesting Category 3 or 4) Care of all newborn infants, including those with potentially life-threatening illness, but excluding ventilatory care and advanced life-support aspects.

___ Class D

Intensive care of the newborn infant, including ventilatory care and advanced life support.

IIIA. Surgical procedures (venipuncture, laceration repair, and incision and drainage of superficial abscesses are automatically permitted):

___ Neonatal circumcision

___ Myringotomy

___ Simple fracture and dislocations

___ Intubation

_____ (Specify inclusive ages)

___ Peripheral arterial cut-down

___ Peripheral venous cut-down
___ Exchange transfusion
___ Umbilical catheterization
___ Other _____

IIIB. Diagnostic procedures:
___ Proctoscopy
___ Subdural Tap
___ Abdominal paracentesis
___ Thoracentesis
___ Bone marrow aspiration
___ Peripheral arterial puncture
___ Bladder tap
___ Arthrocentesis
___ Skin biopsy
___ Laryngoscopy
___ Lumbar puncture
_____ (Specify inclusive ages)
___ Other _____

IV. Pediatric subspecialty procedures (The following pediatric procedures may be routine procedures for a physician trained in a pediatric subspecialty. These procedures may be applied for on an individual basis, if the candidate can supply evidence of training experience and practice utilization of these diagnostic procedures):
___ Renal biopsy
___ Peritoneal dialysis
___ Hemodialysis
___ Pericardiocentesis
___ Cardiac catheterization
___ Lung biopsy
___ Bone marrow biopsy
___ Bronchoscopy
___ Bronchography
___ Hepatic biopsy
___ Ventricular tap
___ Ventilatory care of neonates
___ Vasoactive drug drip
___ Tracheostomy
___ Gastroscopy
___ Sigmoidoscopy
___ Cisternal puncture

___ Myelography
___ Pneumoencephalography
___ Ventriculography
___ Cerebral angiography
___ Intracranial pressure monitor placement
___ Angiography, lymphangiography
___ Chest tube insertion (nonemergency)
___ Endoscopy
___ Other _____

_____   _____
Date of Application   Signature of Applicant

RECOMMENDATIONS OF THE CHAIRMAN, DEPARTMENT OF PEDIATRICS

_____

_____

_____

_____ _____
Date of Recommendations   Chairman, Department of Pediatrics

_____ _____
Date of Approval   Chairman, Credentials Committee

_____ _____
Date of Approval   Secretary, Medical Executive Committee

_____ _____
Date of Approval   Secretary, Board of Trustees

Chapter 5

RELATIONSHIP BETWEEN HOSPITAL-BASED AND PRIVATE PRACTICE PHYSICIANS*

For a number of reasons, hospitals appoint full-time and part-time physicians to practice medicine within the hospital or its outlying divisions. These physicians provide a variety of primary, specialty, and subspecialty services. Among other advantages for hospitals are a potentially tighter rein on quality control and an increased bed occupancy and revenue at a time when financial issues have become increasingly important.

Physicians engaged solely in administration or research rarely pose a problem in the relationship between the hospital and private practice physicians. However, it is more likely that friction (which might adversely affect patient care) may occur when there is overlapping of services provided by the private practice physicians and the hospital-based physicians, whether they are salaried by the hospital or on a fee-for-service basis.

Role of Hospital-based Physicians

Many appropriate roles exist for hospital-based physicians. Certain specialties may advantageously be hospital-based, or regional hospital units are involved. These specialists might include (among others) those involved in burn care, spinal cord injuries, dialysis, cardiac surgery, emergency medicine, pediatric and neonatal intensive care, medical education, radiology, pathology, and anesthesiology. Certain hospital units benefit from continual organization and supervision, which may be best done by hospital-based physicians.

Research and teaching (including primary care teaching) must be maintained in certain hospitals. Commonly these

*Adapted from Committee on Hospital Care: Relationship between hospital-based and private practice physicians, Pediatrics, 75:365, 1985.

programs are centered around hospital-based physicians, although private practice physicians have participated productively in most programs. Teaching and research should not interfere with and, indeed, may enhance patient care when done well.

Within pediatrics, certain subspecialists may best be attracted to a community by an offer of a full- or part-time, salaried position. In this way, the hospital may serve the community by acting as a focal point for recruitment.

Guidelines for Hospital Organizations

The primary goal of the hospitals employing physicians should be to meet the unsatisfied medical needs of the area or community. The private practice community should be consulted in the process of evaluating the medical needs of the community before any definitive action to employ or terminate employment of physicians is taken by the hospital.

Remuneration of hospital-based physicians may be done in various acceptable ways. This is an important and sensitive issue. Ideally, the physician's income should be commensurate with the services provided in the hospital, although it is recognized that several factors influence physicians' salaries.

Granting, increasing, decreasing, or terminating of hospital privileges should be based on demonstrated current clinical competence.[1] The bylaws of any hospital governing admission to the medical staff, delineation of clinical privileges, and access to hospital facilities should be the same for hospital-based and private practice physicians. In the event of termination or alteration of privileges, a hospital-employed physician should have access to due process procedures.

Attending physicians, as well as parents, should be able to choose between available consultants rather than be limited to those employed by the hospital. A hospital-employed physician, as well as a private physician, must never let allegiance to the hospital take priority over allegiance to a patient.

When families initially seek hospital care for their children, they should be apprised of the choices of physicians. It is not appropriate for a hospital to assign automatically the care of a patient to a hospital-based physician if the attending private practice physician has the appropriate privileges to provide the same type of care. For example, a newborn infant should not automatically become the patient of a neonatologist if the patient's medical condition can be managed by a pediatrician appropriately accredited by the hospital. However, an infant's condition may warrant immediate involvement of the neonatologist, either on a consultative or ongoing basis. Assumption of care should be based on the nature of the patient's illness and the knowledge, skills, and experience of the available physician provider. Initial assignment of a patient's care to a hospital-based specialist may be appropriate when the coordinated and complex function of a team of medical care providers is necessary and when the specialist directs that team.

Interaction Between Hospital-based and Private Practice Physicians

Patients are best served by a single physician providing and/or coordinating their care. Any medical care arrangement which unnecessarily interferes with a strong single physician-patient relationship is less desirable than one which does not. At times it becomes necessary to involve more than one physician in a patient's care, but one physician should act as coordinator or director of the medical team. There should be clear understanding of which responsibilities each physician is assuming at any time.

A cooperative, harmonious relationship between hospital-based and private practice physicians is beneficial for patient care, especially in view of the increasing complexity of medical care. Referrals preferentially should be made from physician to physician with appropriate written documentation, rather than relying on communication via intermediaries such as paramedical personnel or house officers. While the patient is under the care of the hospital-based physician, clear communication with the referring physician is vital. Mutual planning for follow-up is encouraged to assure continuity of care. An understanding, give-and-take attitude between physicians is extremely helpful in this team approach to patient care.

Hospital-based specialists generally should assure early involvement of the patient's personal physician (commonly in private practice) in the care of hospitalized specialty patients. This will provide smoother transition in his or her assumption of total care when appropriate (e.g., the newborn infant after recovery from hyaline membrane disease).[2] Follow-up care may be shared by both physicians. For example, the pediatrician may assume responsibility for general health care while other specialists retain the responsibility for care of a certain disease process, such as cancer.

Responsibilities of the Medical Staff to the Hospital

All physicians, whether in private practice or salaried, should be knowledgeable regarding numerous serious problems facing the hospital administration, and they should avoid making demands which are incompatible with current fiscal realities. Certain administrative initiatives and practices, such as the hiring of physician employees, may be threatening to the practicing physician, but it may be helpful for optimal hospital function and economic survival. Cost containment is now a shared responsibility of all physicians, administrators, and patients. Physicians should be encouraged to advise hospital administrators and trustees and government officials about means to ensure quality of care within the constraints mandated by prospective reimbursement, diagnosis related groups, preferred provider organizations, and other new fiscal policies.

Physicians should make themselves available for service on hospital boards and committees to help make appropriate decisions regarding the hiring of hospital-based physicians, other hospital policies, and long-range planning. There should be an equitable distribution of hospital-based and private practice physicians on these committees.

The most important factor in determining the desirability of hospital employment versus private practice should be the ability to serve patients best.

References

1. Committee on Hospital Care: Delineation of pediatric privileges in hospitals. Pediatrics, 70:813, 1982.
2. Committee on Fetus and Newborn, Committee on the Section on Perinatal Pediatrics: Estimates of need and recommendations for personnel in neonatal pediatrics. Pediatrics, 65:850, 1980.

Chapter 6

ADMITTING THE CHILD TO THE HOSPITAL

Parents have become increasingly knowledgeable about the medical and psychosocial support they want for their children. When the quality of medical care is comparable, other factors determine which hospital parents select. For example, parents may ask:
• Do you have preadmission visits?
• What descriptive printed material do you have?
• Is there 24-hour visiting for parents?
• Does the hospital welcome rooming-in for parents?
• Are there designated times for screened sibling visits?
• Does the hospital have a good child life program?
• May I be with my child during procedures and induction of anesthesia?
• May I visit with my child in the recovery room?

Admission to the hospital, either planned or on an emergency basis, is a source of concern for children and their parents. This concern is influenced by the child's developmental level, the nature of the illness and the child's perception of it, and previous experiences with hospitals. Other factors which may be important are language and cultural differences, anxiety levels, coping styles, and the ability to separate and express fears. Family structure, economic status, and emotional climate further affect the child's response to hospitalization.

Preparation for Admission

Four groups share responsibility for preparation of the child and family for admission.

1. The physician, in the office or clinic, should explain the reasons for the hospitalization and provide suggestions for discussion and/or play.

2. The parents should establish a timetable (2 to 7 days) for preparation based on the child's developmental level.

There must be enough time for answering repeated questions and for the parents to convey their understanding and approval of the plan. Parents' information/answers must be honest, factual, and sensitive to the child who does not seem to want to "hear."

3. Books, films, and tapes should be in community public libraries. Children's museums, schools, and other facilities may set up "hospital corners." Some hospitals have successfully used well child visits to the hospital, not including visits to units with patients; others prefer having trained representatives visit classrooms with slides/photographs or tapes and medical equipment for play. Teachers can help a specific child, and through the teacher the class, understand the need for hospitalization.

4. The hospital should distribute written material outlining policies and practices so parents and patients are well informed before admission. Brochures should be prepared especially for adolescents. In addition to the distribution of printed materials, preadmission tours for families should be available and encouraged. A nurse, social worker, or child life specialist may be enlisted to facilitate these procedures.

When there is a spirit of good will and cooperation among these groups, the process is more successful.

The Admitting Process

Ideally, there should be a special admitting area for children. It must be welcoming and have play materials for a wide age group. Privacy is essential for the admitting interview. Admitting personnel should be sensitive to the unique psychologic problems of children and parents, and an interpreter should be available when a language barrier exists. Assignment of one individual to guide the patient and family through the admitting process may enhance efficiency and decrease anxiety.

Tapes, a book, or a board of photographs may be available to help with the transition to the unit. Children and parents should be escorted from the admissions office to the unit.

Nursing personnel should receive as much information as possible on developmental/medical needs ahead of time so they may determine the most appropriate room assignment. A nurse who will be involved in the continuing care should orient the patient and family to the unit. This should include the patient's room, bed, call button, bedside table, toilet facilities, food service, child life areas, and accommodations for parents. The initial tour should not include the treatment room.

The patient should be reassured that a parent will be present whenever possible, and that, when a parent cannot be present, someone else will be available for comfort and support. Nurses, social workers, or child life specialists should be equally well prepared to help, and parents or patients may have a preference. This is a good time to reinforce the reasons parents are given nearly unlimited visiting privileges.

To ensure a smooth process for both children and parents at the time of admission, increasingly hospitals are using alternative procedures:

1. Preadmission tests can be done several days before admission in a clinic, laboratory, or physician's office.

2. Parents may provide demographic and financial information to the admitting office by phone or in the patient's room; similarly, the history of infections, disease contact, immunizations, and so forth may be obtained in advance. (The distress precipitated by repeated requests for histories from parents of chronically ill children requires sensitivity and concern.)

3. Some parents may request that the patient be present when personal information forms (see sample forms at the end of this chapter) are completed, but this can be accomplished in the hospital or at home.

Emergency Admissions

Sudden admissions for illness or injury pose special problems. Emergency admission frequently is confused and hectic, and there is insufficient time for preparation. Nevertheless, the physician should try to answer questions concerning the admission and give insight into immediate treatment plans. Whenever possible, parents and children should be kept together in an emergency situation. It frequently is helpful if parents are permitted to accompany their child to the laboratory or radiology department and even for minor surgical procedures. The emergency room team may work most effectively through a supportive parent.

Hospital Adjustment

Adjustment to the hospital is easier when the child and family are allowed an active role in the admitting process, and when plans are outlined for continuity of care during and following the hospitalization.

Bibliography

For Children and Parents

Althea, Going Into Hospital. Cambridge, England: Dinosaur Publications Ltd., 1981 (available through Pediatric Projects).
Howe, J.: The Hospital Book. New York: Crown Publishers, 1981.
Richter, E.: The Teenage Hospital Experience: You Can Handle It. New York: Putnam Publishing Group, 1982.
Stein, S.B.: The Hospital Story. New York: Walker and Co., 1974.
When Your Child Goes To The Hospital: DHEW Publication, No. (OHDS) 79-30092, Reprinted October, 1979.
Videocassettes: Going To The Hospital
       Having An Operation
       Wearing A Cast
       A Visit To The Emergency Department
Available from Family Communications, Inc. (Mr. Rogers), 4802 Fifth Avenue, Pittsburgh, Pennsylvania 15213.

For Staff

Plank, E.: Working With Children In Hospitals, ed. 2, revised. Chicago: Year Book Medical Publishers, 1971.
Petrillo, M., and Sanger, S.: Emotional Care of Hospitalized Children, ed. 2. Philadelphia: J.B. Lippincott Co., 1980.

Thompson, R., and Stanford, G.: Child Life In Hospitals: Theory and Practice. Springfield, Illinois: Charles C. Thomas, 1981.
"To Prepare A Child," award-winning film available from The Media Center, Children's Hospital National Medical Center, 111 Michigan Avenue, N.W., Washington, D.C. 20010.

Other

Pamphlets: A Child Goes to the Hospital
            Preparing Your Child for Repeated or Extended Hospitalizations
            Your Hospital: Meeting the Special Needs of Children
            For Teenagers: Your Stay in the Hospital
Available from Association for the Care of Children's Health, 3615 Wisconsin Avenue, N.W., Washington, D.C. 20016.
Other information is available from the Association for the Care of Children's Health as well as from Pediatric Projects, Inc., P.O. Box 2175, Santa Monica, California 90406.

Addendum

Pediatric Admission Information

Child's Name _____ Birth Date _____

We want to make your child as comfortable and happy as possible. If we know about his/her nickname, favorite friends, pets, food preferences and above all, normal pattern of living, we can help your child feel more at home. Won't you please help by telling us about your child?

Nickname _____

Parent's name _____

Address and phone number _____

Child's religion _____

Baptized _____ Names and ages of your other

children _____

Does your child need help with dressing? _____ Washing

face? _____ Combing hair? _____ Brushing
teeth? _____Has your child been in a hospital before?
_____.
Does the child know why he/she is being admitted to the
hospital? _____
Does your child seem to make friends with unfamiliar grown-
ups easily? _____.

Eating Habits

Is your child breast-fed? _____ Uses bottle _____ Spoon
_____ Cup _____ Feeds self alone _____ Feeds self
with help _____ If on a schedule, at what hours? _____
What is his/her present formula? _____ What fruit juices
does your child drink? _____ From bottle
_____ From cup _____ Is your child allergic to any
foods? _____
What foods does your child especially like? _____
or dislike? _____
Are there any other feeding routines or aids we should know
about? _____
Is your child allergic to any medication? (please list) _____
_____.

Elimination

Is your child toilet trained for bowel movement? _____
For urination? _____ For how long? _____ Does your
child wear diapers? _____ Does your child use a toilet
chair or toilet? _____ What is the word
for urination? _____ What is the word for
bowel movement? _____ Is the child
taken to the toilet at night? _____ If so, at what time? ____.

Sleeping Habits

Is your child a heavy sleeper? _____When is bedtime? _____ Are naps taken? _____If so, at what time?
_____ Does your child sleep alone? _____ Crib? _____

Bed with sides? _____ Adult bed? _____ Does your child climb out of bed? _____ Describe any special bedtime routine, e.g., having prayers heard, taking teddy bear or doll to bed, etc. _____.

Play

Has your child a favorite toy? _____Did you bring it along? _____ Any favorite names? _____
Is the child used to playing alone? _____ With other children? _____ With grown-ups? _____ Does your child have a pet at home? _____ What is it? _____What is its name? _____.

School

Does your child attend nursery school? _____ Grade school? _____ Name of School _____
Grade _____ Name of best friend(s) _____
Name of favorite teacher _____
List any special interests (hobbies, favorite books, favorite TV or radio programs, etc.) _____
_____
Is there anything else about your child you feel we should know to make his/her hospital stay as pleasant as possible? ___
_____
_____
_____
_____.

Admission and History Screen

Allergies _____
Symptoms of reaction _____
_____

1. Present illness: _____
_____

2. Nickname: _____
   Birth weight (under 3 yr. age): _____
   Where born: _____
   Problems at birth: _____
3. Previous hospitalizations: (location)   Age: Diagnosis:
   a._____   _____   _____
   b._____   _____   _____
   c._____   _____   _____
   d._____   _____   _____
4. Previous surgery: (type)   Age: Diagnosis:
   a._____   _____   _____
   b._____   _____   _____
   c._____   _____   _____
   d._____   _____   _____
5. Usual diet: _____
   Cup: _____ Bottle: _____ Feeds self: _____
   Dietary restrictions: _____
6. Toilet trained: _____ Bowel habits: _____
7. Siblings and ages: _____
8. Immunizations current: _____
   Last TB Tine (date): _____
9. Medicines taken recently: _____

10. Exposure to infections recently: _____
11. Last ate or drank: _____ Last voided: _____
12. Family history   Patient   M   F   S   B   GM   GF   None
    Patient and immediate family:
    Birth defects:
    Blood disease
       (anemia, sickle cell, free bleeder)
    Bone/muscle/joint disease
       (arthritis, MD, fractures)
    Cancer or malignancies
       (leukemia, tumors)
    Lung disease
       (asthma, TB, cystic fibrosis,
       bronchitis or pneumonia)
    Eye disorders
       (blindness, glaucoma, cataracts, eye
       muscle disorders)

Ear problems (deafness)
Diabetes
Heart disease
  (murmurs, high BP, heart attacks)
Kidney infections
  (nephritis, cystitis)
GI disorders
  (ulcers, chronic diarrhea)
Nervous disorders
  (C.P., epilepsy, seizures)
Applies to patient only:
  Frequent infections (throat, ear)
  Childhood diseases
    (measles, mumps, chickenpox)

13. Teaching: orientation to room .... ( )
           explanation of isolation .... ( )
           explanation of test/treatments
           (include I & O, VS) .... ( )
           preop teaching .... ( )
           closed circuit TV .... ( )
           dietary explanations (i.e., tray or not,
           meal times, cafeteria hours, need to ask
           for food/bottles) .... ( )
           directions to emergency exits .... ( )
14. Signature of parent or guardian: _____
    Relationship: _____
15. Physical assessment:

_____
_____
_____
_____
_____
_____

_____
Nurse's Signature

Chapter 7

THE GENERAL CHILDREN'S UNIT

Trends in Hospitalization of Children

The number of children hospitalized and the length of their hospital stays are decreasing. For example, the number of pediatric hospital days per 1,000 population in 1980 was half that of 1970 (Metropolitan Health Council of Minnesota report), and it is likely that this decrease is continuing at the same pace in the 1980's. Third party pediatric patient funding has shifted from the hospitalized to the ambulatory patient, and this development has created an emphasis on outpatient surgery and intensive home care. This decrease in numbers of hospitalized patients, accompanied by rapidly advancing technology, has resulted in a shift to more intensive care for the patients hospitalized; 30% of pediatric patients on medical/surgical wards in 1980 required intensive nursing service, compared to an estimated 5 to 10% in 1973. The current spectrum of ages of children hospitalized for general care is as follows:*

0-1—30%	5-12—22%
1-3—24%	12-20—8%
3-5—16%	

Length of stay in a general pediatric ward is 2.93 to 5.77 days; the average is 3.75 days.

The trend toward reduced pediatric hospital days with increasingly younger patients demanding more intensive care requires

1. Higher staffing ratios for both direct care givers and ancillary support services.

2. Greater space and more equipment for each hospital patient.

3. More rapid turnover of equipment to prevent medical and scientific obsolescence.

*Minneapolis Children's Medical Center.

4. More intensive inservice training for all professionals.

5. Higher ratio of registered nurses to licensed practical nurses and nurses' aides.

6. Pediatric ward design to facilitate constant, close, direct observation by nurses and continuous patient/nurse interaction.

Pediatric Unit Size

The size of the pediatric unit is determined by the community needs. In hospitals with an active pediatric service, the nursing team's methods will in part determine the minimum and maximum size of the units. If several units are possible in one hospital, the children usually will be clustered according to age. In a large children's hospital, they may be grouped by diagnostic category or service as well as by age.

However, many communities that support extremely active pediatric practices do not have inpatient needs that professionally or economically justify a pediatric unit in their hospital, yet the availability of pediatric beds is essential for the community.

Special Considerations for Pediatric Patients

Programming children's hospital care requires knowledge of children's unique health care needs, especially in situations in which special pediatric units are not justified by the numbers of patients; in these situations, creative innovation for sensitive pediatric care is essential.

Relative to health care programming, children are unique in four basic and critical ways:

1. Children are at high risk for death and permanent, crippling sequelae. This is easily understood with disorders limited to pediatric age groups, such as neonatal sepsis, Reye's syndrome, congenital anomalies, or special physiologic handicaps (e.g., limited fluid reserves).

2. Children are in the formative period of life. The impact of this self-evident fact is appreciated by experienced pediatricians, who recognize that many older, physically handicapped patients are unemployable and socially isolated because of their emotional crippling rather than because of their physical impairment. Health professionals now believe children can avoid emotional scarring related to hospital experiences and can even enjoy a significant emotional growth experience in the hospital if the institution demonstrates sensitivity to their psychological status and needs.

3. Children depend on their community for direct health care. The hospital experience may be brief when compared with that in other community environments (family, school, and ambulatory medical care), but a hospital experience is significant for the child and should be planned in coordination with family services and community agencies.

4. Children are dependent on others for funding. Currently, children's special needs are not always considered in general population health funding schemes.

These features that make children unique and different from adults must be recognized for good pediatric program and facility planning.

Planning for Children

The difficult and most important perspectives to include in planning a pediatric nursing unit are those of the child and his or her family. One hospital had 1,000 school children draw pictures of what they liked and disliked about their hospital experience, and these revealed how awesome this experience seemed. Based on the response of these children, the hospital arranged for a playroom instead of a nursing station to be the first area a child encounters after getting off the elevator. The same hospital originally planned a separate rooming-in station; but, based on a survey of mothers, it made rooming-in available in all general pediatric units. Eventually, in response to patient need, rooming-in was extended to all rooms. Patient and family advocacy should be active and effective in designing pediatric units.

Flexibility

There is an axiom related to building: In the planning stage, the program defines the building; after the building has been built, the building defines the program. The current, rapid changes in pediatric practice necessitate that the ultimate in flexibility be designed into the pediatric unit. This can be achieved by building foundations for vertical and horizontal expansion, floor and ceiling construction for maximum vertical flexibility, and wall designs for easy change. The ground floor, which is preferable for a pediatric unit, is most convenient for horizontal expansion.

Unit Design and Communications

The unit design and shape need to promote a therapeutic environment related to children's emotional, intellectual, and physical needs. Continuous visual observation and closeness among patients, families, and nurses provide security, comfort, and safety for the child by facilitating spontaneous, immediate, and informal interaction among staff, patients, and families.

Personnel

Adequate physical facilities can increase the comfort and convenience of a pediatric unit, but the most significant factors in creating an appropriate setting for hospitalization of children are the skill, experience, and motivation of the personnel. To the extent feasible, personnel should be assigned exclusively to the pediatric unit; this will permit the development of the special skills and commitment necessary for the effective care of child patients.

A program of inservice education is essential to instruct all personnel (including housekeeping and administration) in the proper approach and management of young children. For example, a single traumatic experience with an inhalation therapist may undermine the combined efforts of all personnel to reassure and encourage an anxious child.

Nursing

Nurse Staffing Pattern

Because patients in children's units require significantly higher and more intensive levels of nursing care than adults in general hospitals, pediatric services require more registered nurses than inpatient adult units. For consistency and continuity in patient care, a registered nurse should be assigned overall accountability for each patient for patient-family nursing assessment, care planning, delegation of nursing tasks, and coordination and evaluation of the child's nursing care. This assignment assists the child and family to identify "my nurse" and helps personalize the hospital experience. Licensed practical nurses, experienced in pediatrics and supervised by a registered nurse, may be assigned day-to-day care of less complex, less acutely ill patients having fewer problems adjusting to hospitalization. Nursing assistants are best utilized when assigned to a registered nurse who delegates specific tasks in the care of selected patients. Day, evening, and night shift distribution of nursing staff in general pediatrics is approximately 44%, 32%, and 24%.†

The direct care hour requirements for general medical-surgical pediatric patients in a children's unit ranges from 7.25 to 8.35 hours daily per patient, depending on age, intensity of care, census, parental needs, and utilization of support services, e.g., transportation team to take patients to and from other departments. This requirement compares with a range of 16.0 to 24.0 hours per patient in a pediatric life support unit and 15.25 to 17.50 hours per patient per day in a tertiary level neonatal intensive care unit.

Depending on staffing requirements and registered nurse availability, the assignment of patients for nursing care can be accomplished using any one or a combination of several modalities. On larger nursing units (30 to 35 beds), the station may be divided into two or three subunits, each subunit having 10 to 12 designated patients (by room location) and an assigned group of registered nurses, licensed practical

---

†Anderson, A.: Experience at Minneapolis Children's Medical Center. Personal communication.

nurses, and nursing assistants for 24-hour nursing care of the subunit patients. The staff should be assigned to their subunit for a specified period of time (e.g., 4 to 6 weeks) for continuity in the provision of nursing care and development of effective teamwork. The subunit leader (pediatric nurse clinician or clinical nurse specialist) could be assigned continuing accountability for the nursing care of patients-families in his or her subunit and delegate specific aspects of nursing care to appropriate group members. Nursing assistants could be assigned to more than one subunit and/or to housekeeping tasks for the station. Other methods include variations of primary nursing‡ and team nursing, or a combination of primary and team nursing.

Patient Classification

An example of patient classification by intensity of care is given in Table 1, and the distribution of patients by classification at one institution is given in Table 2.

Management engineering techniques (developed by consulting health care management engineers) were used to establish the relationships of direct care hours to nursing interventions. Staff scheduling should be managed to fall within the established ranges.

Unannounced quarterly audits of the unit's staffing experience by an experienced objective nurse evaluator using a patient classification system should be carried out for each shift. A correlation of 90% or better should be achieved between the audit and the unit experience for the same time period. This classification system should be reviewed and updated annually. Once established, the patient classification system is used for daily assignment of patients and is a means of effecting quality control, budgeting, pricing, and planning.

---

‡Primary nursing is a method of having a case manager nurse (primary nurse) provide all nursing services per shift to an individual patient. Team nursing is characterized by dividing services to the individual. The primary nurse develops a therapeutic relationship with the child patient and his or her family.

Pediatric Unit Head Nurse

The head nurse is the pediatric unit's most important leader and resource person. As a role model, the head nurse demonstrates excellence in pediatric nursing, including patient-family assessment and utilization of a holistic approach to family-centered care. The head nurse must recognize the child and family as the predominant figures in planning of care. She coordinates and helps to integrate activities of other services with those of nursing service, and she assures that pediatric unit policies and objectives are in harmony with those of the hospital.

The head nurse initiates and maintains a staff development program to meet the individual educational needs of her staff, including the areas of child development, social-emotional aspects of hospitalization for the child and family, nursing interventions in the medical-surgical management of patient care, and mastery of technical skills.

Nurse Specialist

Pediatric clinical nurse specialists have extensive knowledge of specialty areas and a high degree of expertise in the performance of tertiary nursing care skills. Clinical specialists for particular problems—such as enterostomal care, intravenous administration of medication, parenteral nutrition, and finding new solutions to existing problems—may be effectively utilized in general pediatric and critical care units to improve patient care.

Home care nurses are skilled in making possible the home therapies that formerly required hospitalization (e.g., continuous intravenous infusions).

Physicians

Medical Director of the Pediatric Unit

The proposed requirements of the JCAH state that every inpatient unit "shall be directed by a physician member of the active medical staff who has received special training, acquired experience and demonstrated competence in a specialty related to the care provided in the unit. The director shall have the responsibility for implementing policies established by the medical staff for the continuing operation of the unit, and for making decisions with the responsible physician, for the disposition of patients when the patient load exceeds optimal operational capacity. The director shall assure that the quality, safety, and appropriateness of the patient care services provided within the unit are reviewed and evaluated on a regular basis."[1] A qualified designee shall be readily available for administrative and consultative decisions when the medical director of the special care unit is unavailable. This medical director obviously needs to be qualified as a leader and manager to carry out this designated assignment.

Resident Physicians

The resident physicians are an integral part of the health care team on many children's units, although the attending physician is ultimately responsible for all aspects of medical care. Attending pediatricians of private patients may delegate some responsibility for decision-making and care to resident physicians, but attending pediatricians must continue to maintain personal communication with the family.

Social Workers

A pediatrically oriented social worker should be intimately involved with pediatric patients to serve those with special social needs. Problems requiring social worker support include child abuse and neglect, potentially fatal illnesses, chronic disease, psychologic problems, family difficulties, and economic hardships. Even small institutions should have social workers available to patients and families; larger units often have a social worker stationed on the ward.

Pastoral Care Department

The hospital chaplain may be a full-time, part-time, or volunteer employee of the hospital. The hospital chaplain facilitates the provision of pastoral care by a cleric (rabbi, priest, pastor, or other spiritual person) of the patient's or family's choosing, or he or she may provide the pastoral care personally.

Clerics help parents deal with feelings and reflect on issues regarding their hospitalized child. Clerics will make available to the family such spiritual resources as prayer, scripture, and the sacraments during a time of healing or crisis. The hospital chaplain also functions as a member of the health care team and works with the social worker, nurses, child life specialists, and so forth to provide quality care to patients and parents. Staff support is another important function of the hospital chaplain when he or she is available daily at the nursing stations. Overall, the hospital chaplain's role is to be a visible, available, caring presence; to provide quality pastoral care and counseling to patients, families, and hospital staff on a daily, continuing basis; and to respond during crises.

Parents and Visiting Hours

Parents are urged to stay in the hospital with children who are 6 months to 3 years old to prevent separation anxiety. They are encouraged through unlimited visiting hours to accompany their children to the laboratory, radiology, and for all procedures, including to the operating suite. Parents usually are best able to interpret the hospital and its functions to their children. A therapeutic alliance is established between hospital personnel and parents, and parents are encouraged to take as much control over their child's treatment as is reasonable. This is, of course, excellent training and preparation for home care.

Parents as well as children need to be cared for and supported by the personnel of a pediatric unit. Parent groups led by a skilled nurse, social worker, or child life specialist may be very effective and helpful.

Other Personnel

Described elsewhere in this manual are several other critical pediatric unit functions and personnel, such as child life program, nutrition, volunteers, home care nursing, discharge planning, occupational therapist, physiotherapist, respiratory therapists, laboratory technicians, and pharmacists.

Conferences

Multidisciplinary Committee of the Pediatric Unit

The JCAH also requires that each pediatric unit's activities be guided by a multidisciplinary committee of the medical staff, with the chairman or designated committee member serving as director of the unit. The rapid change in technology and the increasing intensity of care on an active pediatric unit make weekly meetings of this committee a necessity for efficient operation.

Members of the committee shall be the unit medical director (chosen by the hospital medical staff), the unit head nurse, the child life specialist, the social worker, and representatives of other disciplines as needed.

The multidisciplinary meeting agenda usually addresses case study outcomes, special problem issues such as long-term care of children dependent on hospital technology, indications for transfer of patients to other special care units, management of staff stress, needs for inpatient training, effectiveness of child life programs, and behavioral issues related to staff, families, and patients. Plans for the resolution of problems are expedited out of these management meetings.

Individual Patient Care Conferences

Patients with complex or prolonged illness usually require periodic conferencing while the child is hospitalized and at the time of discharge by the professionals whose services are involved. These conferences may need to be held weekly or more often, but they should be at least monthly on long-term care problems. Professionals involved can be the primary nurse, unit head nurse, the primary physician, subspecialists, the chaplain, the social worker, the child life specialist, the teacher, the home care team, and others. The parents, or surrogate parents, also may be included.

The need for these conferences frequently is not understood by many of the key people involved—even resisted by some—so the authority to call them must be given to the unit head nurse and/or the unit medical director.

Financial Counseling

Complex, highly technical pediatric inpatient care is expensive, frequently beyond the reach of family budgets, and requires the utilization of insurance and special funds from private agencies and the government. All these resources are regulated by highly individualized and variable policies for qualification, a fact which makes a professional guide essential for securing the funds to meet an individual child's need. Currently, this service is separate from that rendered by a social worker, whose modern training and experience are in the area of social case work. Financial counselors are now best located through the hospital's credit and collection department, and they are essential for the continuous funding of the care within the pediatric unit. Special situations (defined by hospital policy) require conferencing by the financial counselors with involved physicians and the unit medical director.

Special Considerations for Pediatric Patients

Children's Educational Programs

If children are expected to be hospitalized for 2 weeks or longer, some provision should be made for maintaining their educational programs. Children with handicaps must be considered educable, as though they were not hospitalized but in a residential care institution. Arrangements usually can be made with the school district in which the hospital is located. The use of radio, television, or computerized self-instruction programs to enhance contact with the school system is worthy of consideration.

Meals

Children not confined to bed should be given meals at a table and in a chair suitable to their age and size. A communal dining facility for children not confined to their room simulates eating with the family and may help the patient feel more at home in the hospital setting. In smaller units, the recreational area may double as a dining area. Meals for children should be nutritious, with some allowance made for the child's food preferences. Supervision and assistance must be provided for all preadolescent children during mealtime.

Infection Control

The frequency with which infections and contagious diseases complicate the hospitalization of children requires adequate facilities for minimizing the spread of communicable illness. At least one of the patient rooms should be adaptable for use as an isolation area. The immunization status and contagious disease history of each patient should be recorded at the time of admission. All personnel should be alert to the signs and symptoms of contagious disease, and they should be instructed to report any symptoms of contagious disease promptly to the attending physician.

The hospital's infection control committee should determine policies for isolation of patients or hospital areas and for housekeeping procedures; regulations should be developed for the protection of patients, personnel, and visitors. There is no universally accepted system of isolation techniques, but some form of selective isolation based on the etiologic agent and the method of transmission conserves time and supplies. More importantly, the system must ensure that routine care of the child will not be impaired because of isolation barriers placed between the child and family or hospital personnel. An outline of one generally accepted method of isolation is given in Appendix A.

Architectural Considerations for Pediatric Units

Hospital facilities for children have followed a clear evolutionary pattern in the United States. Early pediatric units were composed primarily of large, open wards. Emphasis was placed on maximizing direct visual surveillance of patients by nursing personnel. These early design themes encouraged social interaction between children, an especially important adjunct to therapy during a long stay.

During the 1950's, coinciding with Hill-Burton funding of hospital construction, standards for hospital facilities deemphasized large wards and favored a liberal mix of private, semiprivate (two-bed rooms), and four-bed rooms. With visual surveillance and peer interaction continuing as high priority design criteria, the four-bed room remained dominant on

2 Bed (Semiprivate) Room

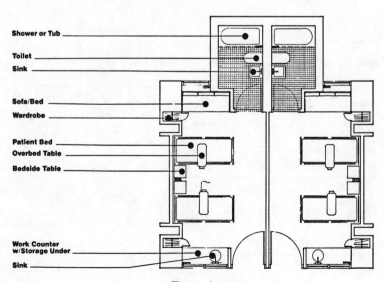

Figure 1

many pediatric units. Children were grouped according to age and/or disease: infants in one room, toddlers in another; or respiratory infections in one room, enteric diseases in another. Depending on the size of the pediatric service of the hospital, many variations of these bed assignment schemes evolved. In general, private and semiprivate rooms were less favored by pediatric nurses and were reserved for isolation or a critically ill child.

The 1960's and 1970's produced dramatic changes in pediatric medicine and a rethinking of facility designs for the hospitalized child. Children were increasingly treated on an outpatient basis for many diseases that formerly required hospitalization. Immunization programs virtually eliminated many childhood diseases. Hospitals with large pediatric units had low occupancy levels. Pediatric units in many general hospitals were either reduced in size, converted to adult services, or consolidated with pediatric services of other hospitals.

With the strengthening of the role of the pediatrician and the pediatric subspecialist, pediatric inpatient units have become more acute care oriented than in past decades. Average lengths of stay have decreased, but levels of severity of illness

4 Bed Ward

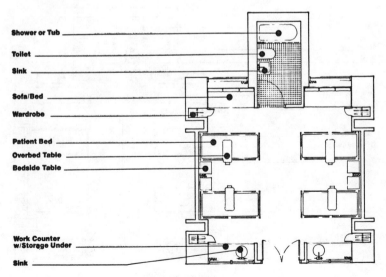

Figure 2

have increased (see pages 72, 73). And a reevaluation of the environment required for the hospitalized child has occurred. Flexibility and infection control have become key concerns. The need to separate children according to medical versus surgical status, according to age or sex, or in response to other criteria has increased.

A dramatic shift from the four-bed ward to private and semiprivate rooms occurred in the 1970's. This change, partly influenced by new hospital design concepts for adults, also was affected by the emerging philosophies of care-by-parent and family-centered care. Further need for change in the design of the pediatric inpatient environment was brought about by recognition that (1) many parents demand the right to be near their sick child, (2) many sick children benefit emotionally and physically from having their parents participate in their hospital care, and (3) the cost of hospital care of the sick child might be reduced with parent participation.

Since the mid 1970's, pediatric rooms have become larger and have moved toward all-private accommodations. The increased size is in response to the increased volume of equipment and staffing associated with the care of the hospitalized child. The larger room also represents an effort to accommodate comfortably the parent who wished to spend significant time at the bedside. These changes, particularly evident in children's hospitals, are somewhat less visible in the pediatric units of general hospitals; because of the repetitive nature

Private Bedroom

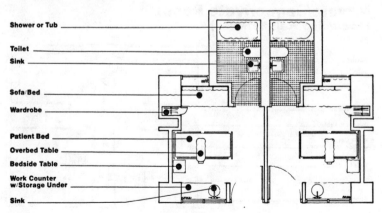

Shower or Tub
Toilet
Sink
Sofa/Bed
Wardrobe
Patient Bed
Overbed Table
Bedside Table
Work Counter w/Storage Under
Sink

Figure 3

of patient floors, pediatric rooms are usually identical to medical/surgical rooms for adults on adjacent floors. Indeed, there are child and family oriented health care professionals who continue to find merit in two- (Figure 1) and four-bed rooms (Figure 2). Private and semiprivate rooms are still occasionally used (Figures 3 and 4, respectively).

Most state and federal codes and guidelines require a minimum of 80 sq ft per bed in rooms of two or more beds, and 100 sq ft per bed in private rooms. The codes and guidelines do not differentiate between adult and pediatric facilities except when describing newborn nurseries. The stipulated area per bed is exclusive of the room's entry alcove, the bathroom, and built-in furniture (e.g., wardrobes) and equipment (e.g., through-the-wall air conditioner units). Many states also specify minimum distances between beds and between a bed and adjacent side walls and foot walls. These minimum clearances are usually 3 to 4 ft on each side of the bed and 4 ft at the foot. To comply with the various space requirements, private and semiprivate bedrooms usually have approximately 170 net sq ft and 250 net sq ft, respectively, or more.

It is a virtual requirement that each patient bedroom have its own toilet and lavatory. To achieve maximum visibility of pediatric patients, many architects are designing the bathroom on the exterior wall of the room; the traditional corridor wall location of the bathroom obstructs visualization of the patient. Each toilet should be equipped with a bedpan

Private/Semiprivate Room
(Accordion Wall Between)

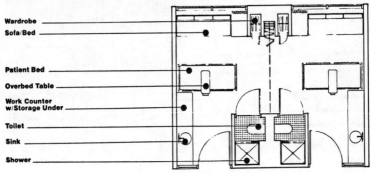

Wardrobe
Sofa/Bed
Patient Bed
Overbed Table
Work Counter
w/Storage Under
Toilet
Sink
Shower

Figure 4

rinser. In response to the recognized importance of regular hand washing by the hospital staff, lavatories are now being placed near the entrance to the bedroom rather than in the bathroom.

Location and number of patient bathing facilities continues to be debated. Although many newer hospitals are planning tub/shower units in every patient bathroom, the logic seems more oriented to overall hospital marketing and image issues than to patient needs. Increasing levels of severity of illness and decreasing length of stay reduce the opportunity for patients to realize the full benefit of a private shower. The alternative, of course, is to plan an adequate number of bathing rooms in convenient locations throughout the pediatric unit, usually at a ratio of one tub/shower per 10 to 12 patients. Shower units *per se* are not appropriate for infants and toddlers, who may require bathing assistance or who may be afraid of the spray. Tubs must be available in a pediatric unit, some elevated for the convenience of the nurse, who often must bathe a pediatric patient.

Providing comfortable accommodations for a parent of a sick child is a simple recognition of a long-standing need. Parents will stay in the pediatric unit whether their needs are provided for or not. The "caring" image of the hospital can be substantially enhanced if a day bed is built in near each patient bed. Several relatively simple, inexpensive day bed designs have evolved; these are more comfortable than chair beds and more convenient than rollaway beds.

Viewing within and between pediatric patient rooms always has been a design requirement that frequently is modified during operation of the unit. Corridor view panels are appropriate for all rooms except those of adolescents, but windows between rooms seem to be undesirable. Patient and parent privacy becomes an overriding consideration, and drapes or blinds usually obscure these windows from one or both sides. Glass view panels in doors to patient rooms may be considered.

Proper lighting of pediatric hospital rooms is an important concern. Inexperienced hospital architects tend to be satisfied with specifying a "head wall" light unit. These units provide adequate general illumination of the patient room, but most do not provide enough intensity for examination or treatment of a patient in bed. Some head wall light fixtures include various types of high intensity, adjustable examination lights as an integral part of the fixture; these units must be evaluated carefully for child safety as well as lighting adequacy before they are used. Alternatives to head wall lighting fixtures are recessed fluorescent lights or recessed high intensity spot lights. Both of these lights are ceiling mounted, are reasonably satisfactory for patient examination, and are out of reach of the patient.

Every pediatric room should have an abundance of electrical outlets plus at least one oxygen and one vacuum outlet per bed. Careful attention by nursing and technical personnel to the location of these outlets will reduce hazards to patients and improve convenience. A nurse call system also should be provided in each patient room. Though younger patients may not be able to use the system, its installation will increase the flexibility of each room to accommodate patients of all ages.

A wall-mounted television is considered a "must" by most pediatric unit planners. The television sets should be out of the reach of younger patients for safety and noise control reasons. In addition to providing entertainment, many hospitals now have patient and family health education programs through a closed circuit television system.

Each pediatric patient room should have flexible storage capabilities. A wardrobe should be provided for patient clothing and other personal effects, and it should be large enough for a coat and other items a parent may wish to store. Provision also should be made for nursing supplies, clean linens, and so forth. Some hospitals prefer a "nurse server" cabinet— a cabinet with access both from the corridor and from within the patient room. These units may offer some convenience to staff but present special fire code problems and reduce the amount of glass possible in a corridor wall for patient viewing.

Planning support areas for a pediatric nursing unit requires an understanding of basic space programming techniques. The size of any room is dependent on "space generators":

1. number of people to be accommodated,
2. numbers and size of major equipment and furnishings,
3. circulation requirements.

The size of a treatment room, for example, must respond

to the foregoing criteria. In addition to the patient, two to three other people may need to be accommodated. The room may include an examination table, one side chair, a 6 ft section of cabinetry, and a lavatory. Access to three sides of the examination table may be stipulated. With this information, a space planner can quickly determine the satisfactory dimensions of the treatment room. Hospital staff should be prepared to discuss their departmental space needs in this level of detail and to supplement room-by-room descriptions with statements of preferred proximity (which rooms need to be close to which other rooms). Hospitalwide systems, such as materials management and cart exchange, also should be considered in space planning exercises.

Table 3 illustrates a "functional space program" for a "typical" 24-bed pediatric unit. Not every suggested room may be necessary in each hospital, depending on total available space on a nursing floor, whether there is an adjacent nursing unit that might share some of the areas such as conference rooms, family lounge, and so forth.

The size of a specific pediatric unit will depend on community need, the existence of competing units, and the hospital's commitment to this service. Individual pediatric unit size can no longer be determined on an emotional or subjective basis. Few units will be permitted to respond to seasonal peaks in demand by having poor occupancy levels most of the year. Currently, planning standards stipulate a minimum occupancy level of 75% on an annual basis.

It is difficult to justify a separate pediatric unit of less than 15 beds or so, except in rural hospitals. For maximum efficiency in the operation of small pediatric units, the unit should be "back-to-back" with another small, compatible nursing unit. This permits sharing of support spaces such as supply storage rooms, conference rooms, and so forth. An ENT unit frequently is cited as being compatible with pediatrics. This arrangement increases the flexibility in use of beds in both units, accommodating occasional peaks of demand.

Unit Configuration

Pediatric units should be designed to maximize nurse-patient visual contact and to minimize distances from the nurses' station to the most remote patient room. The conventional rectangular, double-corridor nursing unit design often accomplishes neither guideline in a satisfactory manner. Although pediatric unit configuration usually is dictated by the shape of nursing units for adults on floors above or below, the architect should be encouraged to adhere to these criteria. It is possible, even in nursing units of up to 48 beds, to limit distances from the nurses' station to the most distant patient room to 60 to 70 ft, well under the maximum allowable of 110 ft. Nevertheless, creative, responsive design efforts are required from the architect.

Nurses' Station

A nurses' station or clerical center should be in a central location relative to patient rooms. In the past, many planners placed the nurses' station at the entrance to the unit to emphasize traffic control. This location often doubled travel distance to some patient rooms and, as a result, became unacceptable.

Some hospital planners continue to debate the issue of open versus closed nurses' stations. The open station maximizes nurse/patient visual contact and direct verbal communication. The closed unit increases staff privacy and reduces distractions and noise. The open unit seems to be more desirable. A compromise solution that includes privacy in the physicians' charting and dictation area frequently is implemented.

A primary care nursing system encourages decentralized charting areas of one per four to six beds. Decentralized charting stations usually are small, recessed counters or desks in alcoves near the assigned patient rooms. A unit secretary usually continues to staff a centrally located "control center." Some planners and architects propose total elimination of the traditional nurses' station in favor of the decentralized areas. However, this eliminates flexibility to accommodate future philosophical changes in nursing team organization.

Appropriate size of the nurses' station and type of equipment are derived from knowing the number of people who routinely must be accommodated. One "rule of thumb" for clerical areas is 60 sq ft per person. For a nurses' station, 60 sq ft per person includes countertop charting space plus required storage for clerical forms and supplies. Additional space should be considered for computer terminals and monitoring equipment.

Physicians' Charting and Dictation Area

A designated area for physicians' charting and dictation should be provided within each nursing station. Usually two to three of these areas are adequate; they may be either a single sit-down counter area, or the counters may be divided to form cubicles which afford more privacy to the individual physicians. Sixteen to 20 sq ft per cubicle usually is adequate and provides 4 to 5 ft of counter space for charts, telephone, and dictating equipment. The physicians' charting and dictating area should be well within the nurses' station. This location strengthens the opportunity for communication between nursing unit personnel and the physician and facilitates locating and controlling patients' charts.

Head Nurse's Office

An office for the unit head nurse or pediatric supervisor should be provided contiguous to the nursing station. A room of 80 sq ft is usually adequate and affords privacy to the nursing manager for employee conferences and other management activities. Typically, the room should include a single pedestal desk and desk chair, a file cabinet or credenza, and two side chairs. This room is not intended for staff conferences involving more than three or four people. However, some hospitals have increased the size of their head nurses' offices to accommodate report and other larger group activities.

A medication room should be located near the nurses' station. This location facilitates control over access to the room and supplies stored therein. Many planners will, in fact, design the medication room so it is accessible only by going through the nurses' station. The appropriateness of this traffic pattern should be considered for each unit to determine if the movement of a medication cart through a clerical area is inappropriately disruptive. Similarly, regardless of the location of the medication room, it must be afforded privacy from distractions that tend to increase medication error rates. Background conversation and traffic of people coming and going through the nurses' station should not be obvious to an individual preparing patient medications.

The size of the medication room typically is adequate at 40 to 60 sq ft. If a prefabricated, stainless steel "med prep" unit that includes a narcotics locker, sink, ice machine, countertop work area, and supply storage is used, it may be incorporated in the smallest of rooms. An additional consideration must be made for the parking and restocking of medication carts that also will be stored in this room. Some hospitals have been reluctant to use the prefabricated medication storage units because of their high cost and have simply adapted standard kitchen-type cabinets. This arrangement usually will consume a slightly greater amount of space with no real compromise in overall function.

Treatment Room

A treatment room is mandatory on a pediatric unit. Many pediatric nurses believe that the patient's bedroom is a "sanctuary" in which invasive or painful procedures will not be performed. Patients' anxiety level is reduced if they know no harm can come when they are in their own bedroom. The presence of the treatment room on a pediatric unit obviates the problem of having adequate lighting in the bedroom, and supplies and equipment are immediately available. The treatment room may be designed with a high intensity, ceiling-mounted examination light and access on three or four sides of the bed. Typically, the treatment room also will include a large section of cabinetry or an exchange cart (either of which should contain special treatment supplies and treatment trays). A hand washing sink, x-ray film illuminators, oxygen and vacuum outlets, a clock, and numerous electrical outlets are all considered essential in a well planned treatment room. Usually, all of these items may be accommodated in a room that is approximately 10 ft by 12 ft.

The treatment room should be located relatively near the nurses' station. This location aids physicians and nurses using the room in obtaining assistance when required, and it improves communication among the staff. A telephone with an intercom system is appropriate in the treatment room.

Utility and Storage Areas

Utility and storage areas frequently are undersized in pediatric units. The variety of supplies, linens, and equipment necessary to support patients of the widely varying ages and sizes routinely found on a pediatric unit must be larger than on adult units. One standard size of linens, typically found on an adult unit, is totally inadequate to meet the needs of pediatric patients in two or three sizes of cribs, youth beds, and full-sized beds. Thus, the ratio of total storage space per patient is generally higher on a pediatric unit.

In planning the size of any storage or utility area, consideration must be given to the type and size of equipment that will be stored in the rooms, the desired circulation patterns, and the number of people who might be in the area at one time. For example, a typical clean utility room, designed around a cart exchange system, may have one large cart for linens, one for central supply items, and one for central storeroom items. The carts must be positioned in a manner to facilitate access to all the supplies stored on them. Doors and aisles must be wide enough to move the carts in and out of the rooms easily. In addition, one side of the room probably will include a limited amount of cabinetry and countertop work space. A one- or two-basin countertop sink is nearly always stipulated for a clean utility room. Under the conditions described here, a multipurpose clean supply room for a 24-bed pediatric unit frequently will be about 160 sq ft.

A soiled utility room frequently will include carts or hampers for soiled linen and for refuse. In addition to these items, the room also will include a clinical sink or hopper and a minimum of 6 ft of cabinetry and countertops with a double bowl sink. Unless large equipment is to be washed in this room, 120 sq ft usually is adequate. If the nursing unit has chutes for soiled linens and trash, it might be possible to reduce the size of the soiled utility room to approximately 80 sq ft.

An equipment storage room is mandatory for a pediatric

unit. A limited assortment of patient beds, intravenous poles, respiratory therapy equipment, and other items may be stored in this room. However, the planners of any hospital facility should not allow nursing units to develop "mini-warehouses." Space on nursing units is too expensive to store idle equipment routinely. Every effort should be made to develop a system, with the housekeeping department and central sterile supply, for the storage and timely delivery of all idle equipment for the unit.

Alcoves should be provided at several points along the corridor in any nursing unit for the storage of wheelchairs and stretchers. It is illegal in most states to obstruct patient corridors with idle equipment. One also must consider the aesthetic aspects of a nursing unit. The typical 8:00 a.m. scenario—patient corridors are littered with dietary carts, medication carts, housekeeping carts, stretchers, wheelchairs, and so forth—is totally unacceptable and hazardous. Every effort must be made to keep idle equipment in a more appropriate location than corridors.

Multipurpose Room

A large multipurpose room, used for organized play activities, patient education, and even group feeding, should be

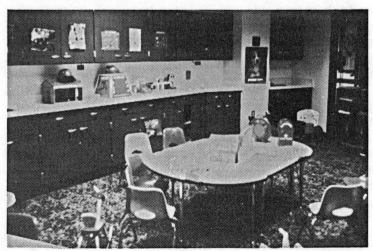

Figure 5

provided on each pediatric unit (Figure 5). This room should include substantial amounts of cabinetry or closets for the storage of recreational and educational supplies and equipment, and a countertop sink area for cleanup. These rooms usually are designed with pediatric-sized tables and chairs. However, if the unit is occupied frequently by adolescent patients, more flexible furnishings or a second room for older patient activities may be considered.

Many planners place a nourishment station immediately contiguous with the pediatric playroom. With this arrangement, it is possible to design a pass-through window between the two rooms to enhance staff efficiency at mealtimes. Although multipurpose rooms rarely are large enough to accommodate the myriad of activities that may be scheduled in them, 300 to 400 sq ft or more are appropriate.

Pantry

A pantry or nourishment station is appropriate for every nursing unit. When two nursing units join in a back-to-back or side-to-side relationship, one pantry may serve both units. Typically, depending on the type of food distribution system in the hospital (i.e., heated cart, heated and refrigerated cart, pellet system, and so forth) more or less space may be required. Many hospitals are now using microwave ovens on individual nursing units and may place the oven on a moveable food service cart or place it permanently in the pantry. It must be placed high enough that small children cannot reach it. The pantry must include an ice machine, a small refrigerator, storage for snack-type items, and a sink. Depending on the food distribution system, space may be required for parking the food service cart in the pantry. Usually a compact pantry of 40 to 60 sq ft is adequate.

Conference Room

A conference room must be available for pediatric nursing unit personnel. This room typically will support the nursing report and continuing education. Two adjacent nursing units frequently will share one large conference room. However, because some privacy for the different teams is necessary during report, the conference room may be designed with an accordion wall in the center to permit dividing the large room into two smaller rooms. Certainly, this arrangement increases the total flexibility in the use of the room while accommodating the needs of individual units. As a rule of thumb, 15 sq ft per person should be allowed; thus, if the room must accommodate up to 20 people on the average, a 300 sq ft space is appropriate. The smaller rooms also may be used for parent conferences, or they may supplement patient recreation or education activities.

Other Facilities

Consideration should be given to whether any other office facilities are appropriate for individual pediatric nursing units. Larger nursing units (i.e., in excess of 30 patients) may justify a full-time child life or recreation therapy specialist. This person should have a small, private office near the multipurpose room. Some pediatric units also assign a social worker full time to the unit. Likewise, this individual should be provided with an office large enough to hold conferences with parents. If the hospital has a policy of decentralized admitting, with the admission function taking place on the nursing unit, consideration must be given to where this function will occur. Sometimes the examination/treatment room is used, or a small, separate admitting office can be planned. Of course, the emphasis in this system is to attempt to reduce the child's anxieties by bypassing the more adult-oriented waiting rooms and admitting offices.

Additional support facilities that might be considered for a pediatric unit include locker/lounge/toilet facilities for unit personnel, toilet facilities for visitors, a visitors' lounge, and a housekeeping closet.

Plans for a pediatric unit within a general hospital not only must include the unique requirements of the sick child and family members but also must reflect the fact that the pediatric unit is part of a larger system. Individual components must interact effectively to enhance efficiency of the entire system. During times of increased competition among hospitals and reduced reimbursement by third party agencies, flexibility and operational efficiency are more important than ever. Organization of a multidisciplinary planning team to assess existing pediatric facilities and plan new facilities is mandatory. The team should be led by a design professional (a qualified hospital consultant or hospital architect) and should include representatives of the medical staff, pediatric nursing staff, other interested professionals, paramedical personnel, and hospital administration. Diverse interests of individual members of the planning team will make consensus building more difficult, but consensus becomes more attainable when objective planning criteria and thorough documen-

Table 1

Patient Classification by Intensity of Care*

Class	Examples of Indicators	Ranges of Direct Care Hours per Patient by Shift†	
I	Child/parents well adjusted. Child independent in ADL.‡ Nurse observes, assesses, and teaches.	Day Evening Night	1.80-2.66 1.43-2.34 0.61-1.11
II	Requires partial assistance in ADL.	Day	2.31-3.48
	Requires feedings at mealtimes only.	Evening	1.85-2.78
	Minimal supervision and/or attention for the child and/or parents re behavioral adjustment. Minimal to moderate supervision for intravenous therapy.	Night	0.87-2.32
III	Requires full assistance with two or more ADL's. Intervention every hour for behavior and/or physiologic adjustments.	Day Evening	2.89-4.19 2.16-3.18
	Nonambulatory with intravenous therapy. Burn debridement.	Night	0.97-1.30
IV	Complex parenteral fluids. Condition unstable. Intervention every 30 to 60 minutes. Death imminent on shift.	Day Evening Night	3.69-4.91 2.72-3.52 1.55-2.05

*System used at Minneapolis Children's Medical Center.

†Professional judgment is necessary in assigning of registered nurses or licensed practical nurses to individual patients.

‡ADL—Activities of daily living: bathing, toileting, feeding, exercising, playing, and so forth.

Table 2

Distribution of Patients According to Classification in a Pediatric Unit*

Class	Percent
I	4
II	36
III	50
IV	10

*Minneapolis Children's Medical Center.

Table 3

Sample Functional Space Program of a 24-Bed Pediatric Nursing Unit

Room/Area	Number of Rooms per Unit	Sq Ft per Room	Total Sq Ft in Unit
Private patient room with toilet/ shower	23	196	4,508
Isolation room with anteroom/toilet/ shower	1	226	226
Nurses' station with physician charting/ dictation	1	160	160
Head nurse's office	1	80	80
Play/activity room	1	300	300
Pantry/nourishment station	1	60	60
Medical preparation station	1	35	35
Treatment/examination room	1	120	120
Clean supply storage/linen	1	160	160
Soiled utility room	1	120	120
Equipment storage room	1	160	160
Stretcher alcove	2	24	48
Family lounge	1	120	120
Conference room	1	150	150
Staff toilet	1	35	35
Visitor toilets	1	35	35
Patient tub room	1	60	60
Housekeeping closet	1	30	30

tation of needs are developed and accompanied by evaluation of planning and design alternatives.

Bibliography

Olds, A.R.: Humanizing the Pediatric Hospital Environment. Hospital Administration Currents, Vol. 25, No. I, January-March 1981, Columbus, Ohio: Ross Laboratories.

Gellert, E., ed.: Psycho-Social Aspects of Pediatric Care. New York: Grune and Stratton, Inc., 1978.

Study to Quantify the Uniqueness of Children's Hospitals. Wilmington, Delaware: The National Association of Children's Hospitals and Related Institutions, Inc., 1978.

A variety of literature is available from the Association for the Care of Children in Hospitals, 3615 Wisconsin Avenue, N.W., Washington, D.C. 20016.

Reference

1. Accreditation Manual for Hospitals (AMH/85). Chicago: Joint Commission on Accreditation of Hospitals, p. 186, 1984.

Chapter 8

THE ADOLESCENT UNIT

A separate adolescent unit, where space permits, is justified on the basis that the care of teen-age patients frequently calls for a staff orientation, management procedures, and facilities unique to this age group. The adolescent unit should be designed and prepared for complicated social or secondary emotional issues as well as medical and surgical problems. Criteria for admission will vary with each hospital. Certain categories of patients, such as those with scoliosis, trauma, and special surgical problems, may need to be in units devoted to these conditions, at least for part of their hospitalization.

Staff

The staff of the adolescent unit should include physicians and nurses who have been trained to provide care for the medical and psychological problems of the adolescent age group. The staff should be familiar with the developmental stages of adolescence and understand how illness may interrupt this process and hamper the achievement of developmental milestones. Therefore, they would be comfortable with variations of adolescent behavior and aware of the teen-age patient's special concerns.

In addition to primary care physicians and nurses, other personnel are important to the adolescent unit. Psychiatric and gynecologic specialists should be available as consultants. Psychologists and social workers should be available to work with the patients and their families. Psychologists are helpful not only for therapy but also in performing psychologic testing. The social worker evaluates the home and assists families with social and financial problems.

An adolescent life specialist should be assigned to the unit to prepare patients for diagnostic and therapeutic procedures and surgery and to coordinate activities which encourage socialization. Because of the adolescent life specialist's non-threatening role, a trusting relationship usually can be established with the adolescent patient early in the hospital course. This relationship can facilitate detection and resolution of maladjustment to hospitalization before major problems arise.

A teacher, appropriate for adolescents who have chronic problems or may be expected to remain on the ward for an extended period of time, might have an office and a classroom within the recreational area.

The director of the unit should be a pediatrician. His or her responsibilities include coordination of the services offered by each of the other professionals on the staff. With the director's leadership, the team should make rounds 3 to 5 days a week.

Quality Assurance

To help assure high quality services, the credentials of all professionals should be reviewed annually by the director of the unit in conjunction with the directors of pediatrics, psychiatry, or other departments as appropriate. A detailed procedure should be developed, reviewed, and "updated" annually, or more often. The medical records should be systematically reviewed.

Guidelines for Adolescent Patients

To help the adolescent patient understand and follow guidelines, rules should be individually explained and consistently enforced. Adolescent patients should be encouraged to become independent, e.g., to trade hospital gowns for their own clothes. Within reasonable hours, friends should be allowed to visit the patient and utilize the hospital's recreational facilities. Staff should be alert to the possibility of visitors bringing in controlled substances. Smoking—both by visitors and patients—although not prohibited, should be discouraged.

Patient's Room

All patient rooms should be arranged on a private or semi-private basis. Patients are assigned to a room according to age so individual roommates will be as close in age as possible. Each semiprivate room should have a bathroom which includes facilities for showering. The room should contain an intercom that may be operated by remote control. The walls of the room and of the adolescent unit corridors should be painted in colors which are appropriate to the age range and similar to colors which might be found in an adolescent's bedroom at home. A double curtain should be provided between the beds in each room and at the head of each bed. Individual reading lamps allow for diffused rather than direct lighting. Access to a telephone is desirable. Although provisions should be made for rooming-in in extreme circumstances, parents should be discouraged from staying overnight.

Recreation Area

A major problem in placing an adolescent patient in a pediatric or adult unit is the lack of recreation equipment appropriate for this age group. Items which could be included in the recreation area are a stereo recorder and record player, video games, television, movie projector, and various books, records, cards, magazines, and current, popular games appropriate to the age range. This would require periodic updating of various items.

An adolescent may enjoy peer support and association in the recreation area and be exposed to therapeutic activities by specially trained personnel, e.g., an activities therapist, art therapist, or child life specialist. Individuals or groups can be observed in this area, and their abilities and interpersonal relationships can be evaluated. The area may be used by adolescents as they see fit within the limits set for the adolescent ward, and it should be their refuge from medical personnel or procedures. In addition to its use as a recreational area, this area also may be used at times by the adolescent patient as a dining room, school room, or conference area. The room should be situated adjacent to a nurses' station for the convenience of the ward personnel as well as for observation and supervision of the adolescents.

Interview/Visiting Room

A room which is comfortably furnished for conversation should be available. In this room, a patient may visit with parents, friends, and other visitors, or simply meditate. The room should be furnished with chairs in an arrangement conducive to conversation; this room will be quieter and slightly more private than the recreation room. It may be used to conduct confidential admission interviews to respect the teen-age patient's need for privacy.

Conference, Examination, and Treatment Rooms

These needs are met with special areas similar to those described for the general children's unit (see page 92).

Snack Bars/Kitchenette

Preparation of an attractive menu for adolescents is important in their care and treatment. A variety of diets (diabetic, weight reducing, low salt) may be required in small numbers for patients in the adolescent ward. A small kitchen should be provided for the preparation of these varied and individual diets. In this area, adolescents could discuss their diet with a nutritionist. This would provide the opportunity for a patient to learn directly the value of a proper diet or gain valuable information in the preparation of a special diet to be continued after discharge. Soft drinks, juices, and prepared snacks should be available during the evening hours. The addition of the kitchen to an area which already includes a semiprivate room, recreational area, and a living-room-type visiting area creates a more home-like atmosphere than the present physical arrangement of most hospital units.

Special Problems

Behavioral issues on an adolescent unit parallel those of the community outside the hospital. Visiting hours may be difficult to enforce; actual practice will reflect prevailing conditions in the specific geographic area. Holidays and weekends pose a particular problem. Some of the visitors may be out of school and not employed, and hence may want to visit for prolonged intervals and interrupt hospital practice. Color-coded visiting passes, a limit on the number of visitors per patient and the length of the visit, and firm but gentle enforcement may help "contain" this problem. Rules for smoking are difficult to enforce unless they are applied to the staff and visitors, and even then they may be circumvented. Prohibition of drugs and alcohol is necessary but difficult to enforce if "recreational" use is widespread in the community.

Adolescent patients may be married or engaged, and enforcement of visiting rules for these patients is difficult. Respect for the dignity and privacy of other patients, the staff, and the unit generally must be achieved by clearly understood rules appropriate to local expectations, and they must be uniformly enforced.

Chapter 9

HOSPITALIZATION OF EMOTIONALLY DISTURBED CHILDREN AND ADOLESCENTS

Pediatric Units

Many children and adolescents in need of hospitalization for psychological or social reasons appropriately may be admitted to pediatric inpatient facilities. However, there are two critical requirements related to the diagnosis and treatment of children with psychosocial problems on pediatric units. First, the medical and nursing staffs must have an interest and expertise in the behavioral aspects of health care. Second, mental health consultants, skilled in working collaboratively with pediatricians, must be available. Their involvement should not be limited to consultation on individual patients; it also should include inservice education for the medical and nursing staffs. If these conditions are not met, admissions of children for psychosocial reasons are generally resented by the staff, and less than optimal care will result. Indeed, the admission of a severely disturbed child or adolescent to a unit with personnel untrained to manage this type of patient and without appropriate mental health consultation can be extraordinarily disruptive to all concerned—the patient, the family, and the pediatric staff.

A pediatric environment may be preferable to a psychiatric setting, if the community does not have specialized child psychiatry inpatient facilities for children. A comprehensive pediatric approach may best meet the needs of emotionally disturbed children with a coexisting medical problem (e.g., ulcerative colitis), when medical management is important (e.g., as in some cases of anorexia nervosa), and when the etiology is in doubt (e.g., as with many children who have abdominal pain).

Suicidal and psychotic children and adolescents and those in need of long-term hospitalization usually are best managed on a psychiatric unit. This is especially true if the child or adolescent is judged to be a danger to either himself or others.

Children frequently are admitted to pediatric inpatient units for "social reasons." An example of this is a child with minimal injuries sustained from an abusing parent, or a child who is neglected by his or her parents. In such instances, hospitalization may provide the child relief from a hostile or neglectful environment. This type of admission also may be resented by the staff, although hospitalization may provide an opportunity to evaluate the family and arrange for long-term care for the child.

Hospitalization often represents a psychologic stress to a child or adolescent, particularly if the admission is for psychiatric reasons. Moreover, disturbed families often may project parental problems onto a child with emotional difficulties, and their desire to hospitalize the child may represent a "scape-goating" of the child. Thus, admitting a child to an inpatient unit should be carefully weighed against other types of intervention, including nonhospital placement of the child outside the home and treatment on an ambulatory basis.

In general, the hospitalization of children with emotional problems does not necessitate special physical facilities, other than an office or room providing privacy and comfort for interviewing patients and families. Children and adolescents in need of a "seclusion room" generally should be hospitalized on a psychiatric unit, although at times it is appropriate to provide a private room and special nursing in a pediatric setting on a short-term basis for suicidal, aggressive, or psychotic children and adolescents. Every attempt should be made not to place children admitted for psychologic reasons in the same room with severely injured or medically ill patients because the ill child's medical condition may cause unnecessary concern and anxiety to the physically well child.

Medical routine and hospital regulations should be flexible to reflect the physical well-being of emotionally disturbed children; they usually do not require daily temperatures or routine determination of pulse rate and blood pressure. Furthermore, they may benefit from outings away from the hospital with parents or friends or from visits home. Procedures for "passes" away from the hospital should be developed in collaboration with the hospital administration, and guidelines should be provided that may be applied to individual patients.

These guidelines should be consistent with fiscal responsibility in that lengthy stays away from the hospital may disqualify time in the hospital for insurance reimbursement. For legal reasons, the leave from the hospital should be recorded in the medical record, including the indications for the leave and that there are no medical contraindications. Parental approval of the leave should be obtained in the form of a signed statement.

Special attention also should be given to maintaining the child's contact with peers and school. Age-appropriate recreation facilities are especially important for children who do not feel ill, and they should be encouraged to wear their regular clothing. Helping the nursing staff with chores frequently is a useful activity. Children with emotional difficulties should not be ignored or "passed over" on medical and nursing rounds, and plans should be formulated in a manner analogous to those for children with medical problems.

Whenever possible, a child psychiatrist should be available for emergency and ongoing consultation. The consultant, optimally, should be Board certified in child psychiatry, and his or her training should have included supervised experiences in pediatric liaison. In many instances, a clinical child psychologist or social worker can fulfill the role of consultant. Mental health consultation is indicated in most instances of suicidal or violent behavior, psychotic episodes, drug overdose, rape, and physical or sexual abuse.

The properly trained psychologist, psychiatrist, or social worker also may be especially helpful in the management of a wide range of nonemergency situations. These would include children with chronic or potentially fatal illnesses, mental retardation, failure to thrive, parental neglect, and psychosomatic problems. There also are frequently significant, long-term, psychosocial and learning problems associated with accidental injuries and severe trauma. Consultation should be requested early to integrate psychological issues into the total care of the child and family and to allow for optimal intervention when crises arise.

Families experiencing the death of an infant from the sudden infant death syndrome may be in need of ongoing counseling, as may the parents and siblings of children and adolescents dying of other causes. Deaths caused by accidents or suicide, especially, may create lasting feelings of guilt and

depression in parents and others who might have been responsible for the care of the victim.

The increasing attention to training in behavioral pediatrics and adolescent medicine highlights the role mental
health personnel have in the education of medical students
and pediatric residents. It is desirable to have these professionals on the pediatric staff and to encourage their complete
integration into the health care and teaching activities of
the pediatric service. Similar involvement of mental health
personnel is indicated in the departments of medicine and
obstetrics and gynecology when these services offer care to
adolescents.

Psychiatric Units

For the acutely agitated, very disturbed child who may be
suicidal or aggressive toward others, a psychiatric hospital
is necessary. There are specialized programs for children and
adolescents with these problems in psychiatric hospitals and,
in some instances, in general or teaching hospitals. In some
states, adequate facilities are available within the public or
state hospital system. However, the majority of communities
do not have appropriate psychiatric inpatient facilities for
children and adolescents, and the pediatrician can assume a
valuable role by guiding the family to the best available
psychiatric unit for their child. Adolescents frequently adapt
well to an adult hospital unit if special recreation and school
programs are available. Hospitalization of younger children
on adult inpatient services is not recommended.

Even when private psychiatric facilities exist for children
and adolescents, the high cost for long-term treatment frequently is not covered by medical insurance. Moreover, the
facility may be outside the local community and necessitate
separation of the child from the family, thereby preventing
a family-oriented approach to therapy. These considerations
must be weighed by the family, ideally with the help of their
pediatrician, against hospitalization on a pediatric ward or
providing intervention on an outpatient basis.

A public psychiatric facility, usually state supported, may
have a "poor reputation" in both the professional and lay

community. It is important to realize that this reputation may be undeserved, and the pediatrician can provide a valuable service to the family by arranging for them to visit the facility under consideration. In the absence of appropriate inpatient facilities, the needs of severely disturbed children frequently can be met, at least partially, by special education programs, good foster care placements, and group homes. School personnel and social agencies can be extremely helpful in arranging such services in collaboration with the pediatrician.

Psychiatric Referrals

Although the pediatrician may not have the training to treat the psychiatric problems that are identified in his patients, he or she can be helpful in the selection of a psychiatric facility and serve as a liaison between the psychiatric staff and the family. Optimally, the pediatrician also can continue to provide the physical health services to these patients and appropriate psychosocial services to the family, with consultation from mental health personnel.

Chapter 10

PEDIATRIC INTENSIVE CARE UNITS*

The second half of the twentieth century has produced an explosion of knowledge regarding the critically ill. The pathophysiology of life-threatening processes such as shock, respiratory failure, and increased intracranial pressure has been explored extensively. Advances in electronic patient monitoring, pharmacology, and improvement in transport systems are only a few of the factors which have drastically changed the nature of critical care.

Simultaneous with the scientific and technical advances has been the evolution of the pediatric intensive care unit (PICU). Children have special medical needs; therefore, it is appropriate that critical care of children be provided by pediatric specialists in units of excellence dedicated exclusively to the critically ill child. There also is increasing recognition of the degree of sophistication implicit in the term "intensive care," which has culminated in the acceptance by the American Board of Medical Specialists of the joint application by the American Boards of Anesthesiology, Internal Medicine, Pediatrics, and Surgery for a Certificate of Special Competency in Critical Care Medicine. Thus, a new subspecialty has been born which reflects the developments in this field.

The following guidelines for PICU should serve as a reference for those wishing to develop new units or to modify existing ones. The contributors to this set of guidelines have included pediatricians, anesthesiologists, specialists in emergency and intensive care, surgeons, engineers, nurses, and child life specialists who focus on the care of children in hospitals. Because of continuing developments in this field, periodic revisions of these guidelines will be necessary. The relative importance of various items is suggested in Appendix B.

For the purposes of this chapter, the PICU shall be con-

---

*Adapted from Committee on Hospital Care and Pediatric Section of the Society of Critical Care Medicine: Guidelines for pediatric intensive care units, Pediatrics, 72:364, 1983.

sidered to be a hospital unit which provides treatment to children with a wide variety of illnesses of a life-threatening nature, including children with highly unstable conditions and those requiring sophisticated medical and surgical intervention. For example, this type of unit would be able to provide care for severe multiple trauma and for patients having open heart surgery. Referral to this unit frequently is the decision of the primary physician.

All critically ill children up to approximately 16 years of age (excluding newborn infants) referred for pediatric intensive care, regardless of subspecialty category, should be placed in units dedicated exclusively to children whenever possible. No attempt will be made to set guidelines for units limiting care to less ill children or for neonatal intensive care units.[1]

General Considerations

An institution providing pediatric intensive care should be a comprehensive child care center capable of providing 24-hour accessibility to a broad range of pediatric subspecialty services necessary for optimal care. The center should be a Category 1 facility as defined by the American Medical Association (see Chapter 14). Critically ill children preferentially should be admitted to these specialized centers. If children must be admitted to an adult intensive care unit, every effort should be made to ensure that medical and nursing care, equipment and facilities, and visiting privileges are appropriate for age.

Effective regionalization of children's intensive care is highly desirable. The special needs of the critically ill child demand a high level of expertise provided by teams of physicians, nurses, and ancillary personnel in sophisticated facilities with special equipment. Not all hospitals, even those treating a significant number of children, will be able to support a fully developed PICU.

An efficient, safe, and rapid pediatric transport system is now practical in all areas in the United States, and its development and operation should be ensured by community health planners. The local PICU staff should participate in its planning and implementation, and it should help ensure that the regional transport system meets the special needs of critically ill children. The PICU staff may participate in the transport of patients as necessary. Effective communication (telephone consultation) from the PICU to the region's emergency medical services system is desirable.

The center should conduct continuing medical education in emergency and critical care pediatrics for primary physicians and other health care providers in the region.

Organization

A permanent critical care unit committee should be established with nursing, administrative, pediatric, pediatric anesthesia, pediatric surgical, and pediatric specialty representation; the committee should include the medical director of the PICU and the unit head nurse. This committee should have medical staff status. There may be advantages in providing the PICU with unit or departmental status and a separate budget. Recommendations for major equipment purchases and for structural and design changes of the unit should come through the PICU committee. The committee should approve and oversee training and continuing education programs for all personnel assigned to the unit. The committee should approve the medical director's position description (including a full definition of responsibilities) and approve the delineation of privileges for physician and nonphysician health professionals. In addition, there should be a written definition of all medical conditions or situations requiring mandatory involvement of the medical director, his designee, or other subspecialists.

The committee should approve policies and procedures such as those pertaining to infection control, pertinent safety practices, traffic control, parent visitation, and admissions and discharges, including triage mechanisms. It should provide for policies and procedures related to monitoring, life-support techniques, and equipment maintenance, including procedures to be followed if essential equipment fails. An appropriate record keeping system should be developed, including provision for periodic review and evaluation of morbidity and mortality, quality of care, and safety.

All members of the hospital medical staff should be permitted to admit patients to the unit if admissions criteria are satisfied and beds are available. The patient's personal physician should be encouraged to continue to participate as a member of the team to further optimal liaison with the family. In certain circumstances, the primary physician may remain in charge of the case as determined by his hospital privileges and local policy. In other instances, he or she may relinquish the case management to appropriate consultants. Ultimate responsibilities always should be clear to all persons involved.

Medical Director

Administration of the PICU rests with the director, who should be a physician with training, experience, and expertise in pediatric critical care. Medical directors for PICU should have completed residency training in a major clinical specialty (pediatrics, anesthesiology, or surgery) and should have had special training and/or experience in the care of the pediatric patient, including advanced skills in monitoring and life-support techniques.

The medical director should assure that certain tasks are accomplished, including, but not limited to, the following: supervision of resuscitation and of basic and advanced life support of all patients; coordination of activities of the multiple services which may be required in a particular patient's care; identification of patients requiring isolation; maintenance, calibration, and replacement of equipment; preparation of the annual budget; organization of education programs for the unit staff; supervision of the collection of statistical data necessary for the evaluation of the unit's effectiveness; implementation of all unit policies and procedures; and coordination of any research done in the unit. In some units the medical director may have attending physician responsibility for all patients, and in others he or she may have the right to request consultation from other physicians or services. A combination of these approaches is commonplace. It is strongly encouraged that the director have ultimate authority over admission, discharge, and transfer of patients in the PICU, especially when resources are limited. Attending physicians should be notified about changes in location of their patients. In the absence of the director, there should be a designee responsible to perform the director's role.

Physician Staff

Physician coverage for the PICU should include 24-hour, in-house coverage by pediatricians and surgeons at the resident or staff level. Every effort also should be made to include 24-hour anesthesia coverage. In addition, a full range of services of pediatric subspecialists should be on call at all times.

Nursing Staff

A high-quality and specially trained pediatric nursing staff with appropriate credentials and demonstrated competence is essential to provide 24-hour coverage. The head nurse should have special training in pediatric patient care monitoring and life support and should be responsible for nursing care, inservice education, staffing, and nursing administration. The head nurse in the unit should work cooperatively with the medical director on all of these activities.

There should be a minimum of one registered nurse per three patients in the unit at all times, with the capability to provide one or more registered nurses per patient as the situation demands. All staff nurses in the unit should be trained in pediatric resuscitation procedures, respiratory care, electronic monitoring, and PICU equipment usage; and they should be able to recognize the psychologic needs of patients and their families. Essential skills also should include the ability to recognize, interpret, and record the often fluctuating signs and symptoms of critically ill patients, to administer drugs and parenteral fluids and electrolytes, and to perform specialized nursing procedures. An adequate period of orientation, including "on-the-job education," should be provided.

Other Team Members

Licensed practical nurses, respiratory therapists, nurse technicians, physician's assistants, emergency medical technicians, biomedical personnel, and various laboratory technicians may provide valuable assistance in the PICU. A unit clerk can handle patient and administrative paperwork and facilitate telephone communications and record handling.

Other staff may include a variety of nurse specialists, child life specialists, clergy, social workers, physical and occupational therapists, and nutritionists. There also must be adequate administrative staff. Appropriate job descriptions should be generated for all personnel.

Teamwork is essential for the management of the critically ill child. The effectiveness of the team at the bedside depends on the technical skills and competency of each member; appropriate attitudes and mature behavior also are required. Communication among all members of the team is imperative. Attention should be given to the effects of stress on team members. Support by the chiefs of departments is essential. Patient care must be guided by written policies and procedures.

Other Support Functions

Laboratory services should be available on a 24-hour basis, including microspecimen chemistry techniques, blood gas determinations, radiology, blood bank, and pharmacy services.

Physical Characteristics—External

The PICU should be a geographically distinct unit within the hospital, with controlled access. It should be located adjacent to or within direct elevator travel to the emergency room, operating room, recovery room, and laboratory and radiology departments. It may be advantageous for critical care units to be close to each other. A physician's on-call room should be close by, as should the director's and head nurse's offices. No traffic to other departments should pass through the PICU. Supply and professional traffic should be separated from public and visitor traffic, if possible. Adjacent elevators should have key control.

A waiting room for families should be provided nearby, ideally including arrangements for sleeping. In addition, a space for family counseling is essential.

Other facilities located nearby should include a staff lounge and personnel locker space. Sufficient storage space for equipment, janitor's supplies, linen, and patient belongings is important and should be planned to allow for increasing needs. A nourishment station and clean and soiled workrooms should be close by.

An intermediate care area adjacent to the PICU is desirable and allows for the continuing care of the patient as he or she recovers. Because of the close association of intermediate care areas to the PICU, it is recommended that both units be administered by the same personnel.

Physical Characteristics—Internal

The ideal size for a PICU is unknown. Units smaller than approximately six beds risk inefficiency, and units larger than approximately 16 beds may be difficult to manage unless they are appropriately subdivided.

Isolation rooms with separate washing and gowning facilities should be provided within the intensive care unit for critically ill patients who may be infected or who are at increased risk for nosocomial infection. In addition, each patient should be allowed a modicum of privacy via curtains when necessary.

A central station serves the functions of information exchange and communications center. It is helpful if patients are directly visible from the central station. Central electronic patient monitoring may be utilized but does not substitute for bedside observation. A computer/microprocessor is highly beneficial. There should be a medication station with a drug refrigerator and narcotics cabinet. A separate charting area for physicians and nurses allows for undisturbed thinking. A conference room nearby allows for teaching, conferences, and counseling. There should be adequate working and charting space, shelf space, drawers and cupboards for individual supplies, and appropriate mechanisms for hanging of intravenous fluids. A hand washing lavatory should be near each patient's bedside. Staff and patient toilets should be provided. There should be a mechanism for summoning additional personnel from the PICU to the bedside in an emergency, and a hospitalwide system. Provision for administration of inhalation anesthetics within the unit may be appropriate in some settings.

The presence of windows and clocks allows for day-night orientation. Television sets, mobiles, decorations, and attractive colors may provide some distraction for the child. Designs on ceilings may be helpful for children who must lie on their back.

The bedside arrangement of equipment should provide for complete accessibility to the patient. For resuscitation, access to the patient's head and neck is imperative, and there must be sufficient floor space to assemble the necessary personnel and equipment. Each bedside must be provided with the appropriate electrical, illumination, gas supply, and vacuum outlets (see Appendix C).

The PICU should have appropriate heating, ventilating, plumbing, and air-conditioning facilities as well as relevant fire safety features. Various local and federal codes govern these factors (see Appendix C).

Portable and Emergency Equipment

The equipment necessary for emergency or continuing care must be readily available to the patient and, if not affixed at the bedside, must be portable and easily brought to the child. Appendix B includes a listing of some items available at present, but it is not necessarily complete. All equipment should be serviced on a regular and frequent basis to ensure good working order. (See also Resuscitation Cart Supplies, Appendix D.)

Physiologic Monitoring

Extensive physiologic monitoring is one of the hallmarks of the PICU. Basic monitoring capability should provide for ready determination of weight, blood pressure (by sphygmomanometer, Doppler ultrasound, oscillometry, or intra-arterial cannulation), temperature (including capacity to measure extremes of hypo- and hyperthermia), heart rate, electrocardiogram (continuous wave form), and respiratory rate and corresponding wave form. Central venous, pulmonary artery, intracranial, and esophageal pressure monitoring with display of corresponding wave forms should be available. A mechanism for simultaneous measurement of three or more pressures is necessary. All pressure, heart rate, and respiration monitors should have high-low visible and audible alarms. Availability of hard copy of all wave forms is helpful. Appropriate electrical safety provisions should be assured to protect the patient (see Appendix C). It may be advantageous to have monitoring equipment which is interchangeable with that in other units of the hospital.

Cognizance should be taken of the development of monitoring capabilities, including continuous EEG monitoring, mass spectrometry, end tidal PCO_2, transcutaneous oxygen and carbon dioxide tensions, continuous monitoring of pulmonary function during artificial ventilation, and evoked brain stem potentials. These techniques are likely to become more widespread in the next decade, as is an increased sophistication in the use of the data generated via telemetry, trend analysis, and computerized display of multiple physiologic variables. Computerized feedback mechanisms are being developed and will be important in the near future. There should be long-range planning for use of such equipment as it becomes available and practical.

Availability of biomedical engineering resources to the PICU is becoming extremely important. In addition, 24-hour availability of maintenance services or interchange for all biomedical equipment is mandatory. All PICU equipment should be tested for safety and proper function by a qualified person and retested at least quarterly, with records kept.

Child Life and Family Concerns

Parents should be allowed to stay with their critically ill child as much as possible. The familiar face and voice of a parent may reach a child who appears comatose but is beginning to respond to stimuli.

For both parents and staff, it is extremely important to keep the atmosphere positive, pleasant, and as much removed from the feeling of hopelessness as possible. Parents' alertness and emotional control play a major role in a successful unit; therefore, the PICU staff should encourage parents and relatives to get proper rest and nutrition during times of crisis when they may neglect themselves. One person should assume responsibility to be the chief source of medical information and have regular contact with the parents. If this person is a house officer, it should be made clear that the discussions are made under the direction of the attending staff physician.

The waiting area close to the unit should be used for parents to repose and try to gain self control. Emotions which might upset children or other parents may be appropriately displayed in this area. Some children, even though receiving intensive care, still may be exposed to the environment of play provided by toys available in the PICU. Parents should be encouraged to interact with their children, using familiar toys or other objects to simulate a home environment. Child life specialists can be extremely beneficial and should become well acquainted with the child.

The intensive care unit should have personnel available who have responsibility for the emotional and psychologic aspects of the child and family but do not have formal medical responsibility for the patient. Such professional persons as child psychiatrists, social workers, pastoral care specialists, and child life specialists should have knowledge, tact, and empathy; and they should be available for consultation with the family whenever special emotional support is needed. These specialists may help improve the communication between medical and nursing staff and the family.

Reference

1. Committee on Fetus and Newborn and Committee on Obstetrics: Maternal and Fetal Medicine: Guidelines for Perinatal Care. Evanston, Illinois: American Academy of Pediatrics, and Washington, D.C.: American College of Obstetricians and Gynecologists, 1983.

Chapter 11

SURGICAL SERVICES

The provision for adequate surgical services is an important endeavor of any hospital caring for children. Over one-half the children in hospitals have been admitted for consideration of diseases which may require surgery or for surgical procedures. Thus, a large proportion of hospital care of children is devoted to "surgical patients." Among the challenges inherent in providing adequate surgical services are the extensive variety of childhood disease processes and the differing requirements for care of routine or complex and critical pediatric surgery patients. The appropriate management of these facets of pediatric care is important to any hospital caring for children.[1]

Administration of Surgical Services

Competent, effective delivery of surgical services is enhanced when a committee for surgical services can be assigned such a responsibility. This committee will require representation from the surgical specialties, from pediatrics, and from the hospital administration. The committee's principal activities are the delineation of surgical privileges, the assessment of hospital capability, and the promotion of effective working relationships among physicians. Each of these activities needs to be managed in accordance with and coordinated with general hospital policy, as detailed elsewhere in this manual.

Each hospital must evaluate the qualifications of its member physicians. Guidelines available to hospital committees to help in determining expertise in caring for children include the following:

1. Specific certification in a child subspecialty—an example is the Certificate of Special Competence in Pediatric Surgery awarded by examination by the American Board of Surgery.

2. Membership in organizations indicating a physician's in-

terest in children's surgery. Examples are the Academy's Sections of Surgery, Orthopedics, or Urology.

3. A practice profile indicating a considerable and successful experience with specific pediatric surgical procedures.

The committee for surgical services may define the hospital's surgical capabilities. This definition should indicate the areas of surgery in which the hospital facilities and personnel are competent. Areas for consideration include the availability of ancillary, anesthesia, laboratory, and radiology services appropriate for infants and children. The performance of surgery implies the availability of medical and surgical pediatric subspecialty support and consultation, such as to ensure adequate preoperative patient preparation and suitable management of complications inevitable (or unavoidable) with particular surgical procedures.

The committee for surgical services can contribute much to promote an effective working relationship among the physicians caring for surgical patients. No child undergoing surgery should be deprived of the general and developmental expertise of the pediatrician, nor of the specific knowledge and techniques of the surgeon.

Facilities

Operating Room

The general requirements for an operating room for children's surgery are met by an adequate adult facility. However, optimal surgical management of infants and children requires specific attention to details of operating room construction, equipment, and surgical scheduling. Appropriate intraoperative care of infants and children is enhanced by the availability of an operating room with heating and cooling capability to maintain an ambient temperature of up to 85°F (30°C), with humidity appropriate for the temperature selected. Operating room equipment should provide for thermal maintenance and for thermal and cardiac monitoring of patients. Instrumentation appropriate for specific operative procedures in infants and children is necessary. Children, particularly infants, have diminished nutritional and metabolic reserves with a high metabolic rate, and infants have a high thermal neutral zone.[2] Children and infants tolerate delays in diagnosis and treatment less well than adults. Therefore, preferential elective scheduling of children and infants is desirable to ensure a predictable and optimum time for surgery. Operating room personnel familiar with infants and children, and specifically assigned to children's surgery, can minimize the impact of these physiologic differences.

Postoperative Recovery Room

Children usually can be expected to recover well from anesthesia and surgery. Both surgery and anesthesia customarily will have been relatively brief; and, in children, preexisting organ system disability frequently will be minimal. Two special concerns of the children's postoperative recovery room are those of cardiac and respiratory function and the maintenance of thermal stability and conservation. Management in these areas requires personnel familiar with and comfortable in observation, assessment, and intervention in the postoperative child. Physician availability, preferably that of an anesthesiologist expert in children's care, is desirable.

Ambulatory Surgery

Ambulatory surgery done in free-standing centers or in ambulatory units within hospitals is of increasing importance in children's surgery. From 20% to 50% of operative procedures in children can be done on such a basis. Ambulatory surgery has been found applicable in a variety of children's surgical specialties, including general pediatric surgery, orthopedic surgery, urology, dentistry, otorhinolaryngology, and plastic surgery. When properly monitored, ambulatory surgery is safe, cost-effective, and minimizes the effects of family separation and dislocation. The prerequisites for safe ambulatory surgery are the following:
1. Healthy children not requiring extra care or evaluation

and with the expectation of adequate operative compliance.

2. A defined procedure of modest magnitude with a low complication rate and a minimal rate of needed postoperative hospital admission (not to exceed 1%). Tracheal intubation, of itself, is not a contraindication to ambulatory surgery.

3. A procedure not needing complicated postoperative care.

4. A procedure requiring no unusual postoperative restriction of activity.

The specific procedures to be done in a hospital on an ambulatory basis need to be considered through conference of the committee for surgical services as well as representatives of anesthesiology, surgical subspecialties, and hospital administration. Ambulatory surgery necessitates a short period of pre- and postoperative observation. The management of the ambulatory surgical patient and his or her family should be systematized to ensure adequate and effective preoperative counseling and postoperative instruction. The specific topics of instruction include precise details of preoperative preparation, including the length of preoperative fasting, the clothing and equipment to be brought with the patient, instructions regarding postoperative activity, and details of the postoperative observation and management which are to be provided by the family.

Nursing Units

The pediatric surgical patient, whether in a general hospital or a children's hospital, requires experienced, compassionate nursing care. This is enhanced by clustering or consolidation of patients, which permits concentration of appropriately qualified personnel. This clustering also will facilitate optimal utilization of available equipment and supplies. In the general hospital, this aim frequently will be met by two combined pediatric/pediatric surgical units. Hospitals choosing to care for newborn infants or critically ill children will find it desirable to provide the specialization of personnel and space afforded by a neonatal nursery and an intensive care unit. In the children's hospital, a clustering of surgical patients by disease or specialty should be considered. Although separation by age of patient may be desirable, expert care of patients is enhanced when patients with similar illness are grouped for maximal utilization of available nursing resources. Family support and cooperation, as well as the child's psychological well-being, can be encouraged by the provision for parent or family rooming-in. Rooming-in is particularly effective for the surgical patient because of the positive effect of family participation in specific activities of recovery.

Surgical Nursing Personnel

Surgical nursing of pediatric patients is a subset of both pediatric and surgical nursing. Ideally, personnel are educated in and comfortable with both types of nursing endeavor. This admixture does not appeal to all nurses, and personnel should be encouraged to self-select this group of surgical patients. Self-selection plus the clustering of surgical patients will provide the framework for adequate experience in pediatric surgical nursing. This specialization, whether it is pediatric/pediatric surgical nursing in the general hospital or surgery specialty nursing in a children's hospital has the additional value of defining a specific group of nursing personnel to whom inservice educational efforts can be directed.

The nursing requirement for a pediatric surgical unit is comprehensive, 24-hour nursing by personnel familiar with age-dependent disease processes, their complications, and their pre- and postoperative management. Specific skills required of the pediatric surgical nurse are those of airway management, monitoring equipment, intravenous therapy for the infant and child, and mastery of the use of tubes, dressings, and drains as determined by the patient's disease and surgical procedure.

References

1. American Pediatric Surgical Association, Committee for Standards of Care for Pediatric Surgery: Standards of care for pediatric surgery. Unpublished manuscript. 1979.
2. Rowe M.J., and Marchildon, M.B.: General Principles. *In* American College of Surgeons: Manual of Preoperative and Postoperative Care. Philadelphia: W.B. Saunders, pp. 281-285, 1983.

Chapter 12

ANESTHESIOLOGY SERVICE

The primary goal of the pediatric anesthesiology service is to contribute to the optimal health care of infants, children, and adolescents. The service may be comprised of a cadre of anesthesiologists and nonphysician anesthetists (with defined medical supervision and direction) dedicated to providing anesthesia for children. To meet this goal, anesthesiology service personnel require specialized interest, aptitude, training, and experience in the care of children. Skills required for safe anesthetic management are based on knowledge of physiology, pharmacology, monitoring modalities, specialized equipment for anesthetic administration, and equipment and techniques for airway management which have specific pediatric application.

The usual care of the infant or child scheduled for anesthesia should include preoperative evaluation of the child's physiologic and psychologic status. Following preoperative chart review, history, and physical examination, the anesthesiologist discusses with the child and parents the anticipated plan for anesthesia, including premedication, induction technique, and anticipated aftereffects. Informed consent, specifically for anesthesia, is best obtained by anesthesia personnel from parents rather than being included in a blanket authorization for hospitalization or surgery. Intraoperative management of the anesthetized child must include the ongoing evaluation and maintenance of fluid, electrolyte, and metabolic requirements, and adequate monitoring, surveillance, and support of the vital functions of the unconscious and sometimes critically ill patient. Postoperative care of the child includes supervision during the recovery room stay until the child's care is transferred to other appropriate personnel. The postoperative care of the child also includes follow-up visits to assess the physiologic and psychologic impact of the anesthetic and perioperative events.

To document the satisfactory provision of surgical anesthesia services to the patient, the anesthesiology service is responsible for quality assurance. The first element of quality assurance should be a delineation of the requirements for pediatric privileges for physician and nonphysician anesthetists. These privileges should be based on the individual's education, clinical training, experience, and demonstrated skills. Evidence of continuing quality assurance may be provided by mechanisms including periodic audits of patient care with subsequent follow-up action, morbidity and mortality conferences, documentation of continuing education of service personnel, and participation in other institutional quality assurance and educational programs. The anesthesiology service should have written policies and procedures regarding patient care as well as safety regulations concerning the operating room environment and anesthesia equipment.

The anesthesiology service also may provide valuable clinical support and leadership in patient care areas outside the operating room. These may include respiratory therapy, intensive care, ambulatory or day surgery, and training and execution of cardiopulmonary resuscitation. For day surgery procedures, the anesthesiology service may assume a major role in appropriate patient selection and the determination of their appropriate preoperative acute clinical status. Postoperative responsibility may be extended to include a discharge order from the outpatient facility. Postoperative follow-up evaluations and quality assurance assessment should be carried out in the same manner as performed for regular inpatient anesthetic procedures.

As part of a hospital's policy making and governance process, the anesthesiology service may make substantial contributions to appropriate committees dealing with the overall medical staff supervision, acquisition and approval of new drugs or medical devices, and development of environmental, electrical, or atmospheric safety standards.

Anesthesia departments in pediatric hospitals may serve as an educational resource for affiliated university or hospital anesthesia training programs. This activity should be encouraged as a method of stimulating the interest of internal staff and as an avenue for providing appropriate training to facilitate subsequent pediatric care by anesthesia practitioners in the community hospital setting.

Clinical research is a logical extension of the activities of an anesthesiology service committed to excellence in patient care and education. Resources and feasibility for research will vary substantially from one setting to another. Investigational projects (screened and monitored by appropriate review committees when human subjects are involved) should be encouraged.

Policies regarding parental visits during induction of anesthesia and in the recovery room should be flexible, depending on the facilities available, attitudes of the personnel, and the families' wishes. In some instances, these visits may be beneficial, but the decision of the hospital and medical staff should be based on the realities of each situation.

Chapter 13

AMBULATORY PEDIATRIC SERVICES

The size and range of ambulatory services for children is based on the needs of the community which the clinic or hospital serves. Urban hospitals serving patients of low socioeconomic status may require ambulatory care services with considerable space and patient volume relative to the inpatient services. Teaching hospitals usually have clinics in most pediatric subspecialties. However, in communities with many private practitioners, the hospital will be used primarily for inpatient care, with only limited ambulatory services. However, many basic goals of ambulatory care in a community hospital are comparable to those of teaching institutions.

The objectives of a comprehensive pediatric ambulatory service include the following:

1. Provision of appropriate initial care and advice for children with any health problem, including (a) identification and prompt initial management (with appropriate referral) of life-threatening illness or injury and (b) immediate management of the more common or uncomplicated minor medical and surgical child health problems, as well as appropriate reassurance and education of the patient and family.

2. Management of complex, recurrent, and chronic health problems of children, with guidance from consultants when appropriate.

3. Provision of health maintenance services to children and their families, including (a) immunization and similar preventive measures, (b) early identification of health problems and risk factors, (c) education and counseling regarding health and development, and (d) appropriate support and guidance of the family with emotional problems and of children who have chronic illnesses or special problems.

4. Identification and utilization of community resources to extend social, financial, and medical services to children and their families.

Organization

A pediatric ambulatory service may be organized into several subdivisions.

General Medical Clinics

Nonscheduled Clinics

The nonscheduled clinics provide primary care for children with episodic problems who otherwise might come to the emergency room. Because these clinics provide only acute episodic care, children requiring extended follow-up or health supervision should be referred to one of the other clinics.

The nonscheduled clinic should be open during daytime hours; evening and weekend services may be necessary, depending on need and the availability of personnel. In general, the hours of operation should be geared to the needs of patients. The staff should consist of pediatricians and/or pediatric nurse associates, with consultants representing the various subspecialties on scheduled call. This type of clinic is a preferable alternative to the inappropriate use of an adult- or trauma-oriented emergency department, especially if qualified pediatricians are not included in the emergency department staff.

General Medical (Continuity or Scheduled) Clinics

The scheduled clinics provide pediatric care for conditions not requiring subspecialty consultation and for which prevention and education must be emphasized (e.g., diabetes, asthma). Patient visits are by scheduled appointment. Hospitals, particularly in urban settings, also may provide primary health care to a defined population of children who have no other source of care. In some settings, continuity clinics should be organized as a private practice to the extent possible, with emphasis on growth, development, parent and child health education, and a stable, professional-patient relationship. The clinic may be staffed with pediatricians and pediatric nurse practitioners, and it is valuable for training of house staff in the natural history and management of chronic disease. House staff is best assigned on a scheduled, long-term (1- to 3-year) basis if continuity is to be achieved. This experience is considered an important, if not essential, part of residency training. Social workers, health educators, and child life specialists are invaluable adjuncts to these clinics.

Specialty and Subspecialty Clinics

Specialty and subspecialty clinics are designed for children with specific health problems, usually limited to an organ system or disease process. Some general pediatric care also may be provided. Children with chronic diseases requiring periodic expert consultation may be followed in these clinics, although the patient may receive routine care from a private practitioner or a general medical clinic. Depending on the specialty, these clinics have varying needs for space, staff, and equipment. Visits are almost always by scheduled appointment.

Chronic Care Clinics

Certain special problems (e.g., cleft palate, myelodysplasia, certain collagen diseases) are best managed in a multidisciplinary clinic. Teams of specialists often provide more efficient and more effective care, particularly if management is coordinated by a single individual. The care rendered should be comprehensive and generally requires the additional services of social workers, health educators, physiotherapists, and nursing care specialists.

Home Care

The clinic may provide care and support services in the

home to ensure continuity and to reduce the number of hospitalizations or outpatient visits. Such outreach programs require close cooperation and coordination with community services such as departments of public health, visiting nurse associations, and other voluntary health agencies.

Adolescent Health Care Clinics

The adolescent health care clinic may provide care and support services to individuals between 12 and 21 years old. These clinics should be staffed by medical and nursing specialists in adolescent health care. Counseling support services and adolescent mental health consultants are valuable adjuncts.

Pediatric Ambulatory Surgery Clinics

The ambulatory surgery clinic may provide care and support services to children who may benefit by a reduced hospitalization or by ambulatory surgery. This type of clinic requires the services of pediatric nurse associates/specialists.

Clinic's services should be available 24 hours a day, usually by arrangement with a specified service (on-call physician or emergency department) for patient care outside the clinic's operating hours.

Personnel

A Board-certified or Board-eligible pediatrician should direct all ambulatory services for children. This individual is accountable for policies, procedures, and management of the department. Physicians trained in pediatrics and/or pediatric nurse practitioners provide individual patient care according to established policies, under the supervision of the director.

Clerks, receptionists, and nurse aides, responsible to the

head nurse, relieve professional medical personnel of administrative and other nonmedical duties (e.g., reception and registration of patients, completion of forms, patient transfers, telephone answering, and temperature and body measurements). Bilingual or multilingual personnel are mandatory in clinics serving foreign-language-speaking populations. Medical social workers assist in dealing with the many social and environmental problems of illnesses. Social workers may be based full time in the ambulatory pediatric department or assigned as needed by the social services division of the hospital. The following may be helpful in estimating personnel requirements for delivery of ambulatory care:

- chief clinic nurse, who is a registered nurse;
- registered nurses: 1/10,000 annual visits;
- pediatric nurse practitioners for well child examinations and health maintenance activities: number should not be based on number of visits but rather on the scope of services provided;
- licensed practical nurses: 1/5,000 annual visits, depending on services provided;
- receptionist: one;
- clerks: three to four, depending on number of visits;
- social service workers by assignment as required;
- community health aides: 1/10,000 visits;
- child life specialist, especially for waiting area, in large clinics;
- bicultural, bilingual translators trained in medical terminology, when appropriate.

Facilities and Equipment

General

Children ideally should be examined and treated in facilities separate from those of adults. If the same area must be used, pediatric and adult activities should be conducted at different times. Likewise, adolescents should be scheduled during a separate time period from those for either adults or younger children. The waiting room requires more space than for a comparable number of adult patient visits because children invariably are accompanied by other family members. Sick children should be separated from healthy ones during the waiting process.

Thoughtful design of waiting rooms for children may help to diminish anxiety and apprehension in young patients and their parents.[1] Children need to feel comfortable and self-controlled, and to be purposefully active. Three important features of waiting room design are the position of major transit zones, the arrangement of seats, and the location of play space.

A single path entry-to-reception-to-exit maximizes the space available for seating and play. Although the most efficient arrangement involves placement of the receptionist near the entrance, small intimate rooms may provide a more confidential atmosphere for obtaining initial personal information.

The seating area may be made more comfortable by creating clusters of chairs in L-shaped configurations rather than lining them along a wall. A play area should be located away from the traffic zone, with play and sitting areas, storage and display facilities, and a milieu which encourages children to explore and use toys, crafts, games, and other materials appropriate for various ages.[1] A family/child education area with health promotion/information materials should be provided.

A system of large directional signs helps guide parents, especially those visiting for the first time. Signs often must be bilingual. A system of colored lines embedded in the floor or along the walls, with each color leading to a designated area, is effective in directing parents, especially if illiterate, through the ambulatory department.[2]

Patient flow is facilitated by provision of a separate room for weighing, measuring, and other screening procedures.

Examining rooms should reflect the needs of children and provide sufficient space for the child, parents, a physician, and a nurse. A minimum of 80 to 100 sq ft is recommended. A sink, examining table with a step stool, a chair and a writing surface for the physician, and chairs for the parents are minimal requirements. Necessary examination equipment (e.g., otoscope, ophthalmoscope, and sphygmomanometer) may be wall mounted or portable and located out of reach and sight of small children.

Selection of wall colors depends on local preference and the amount of natural light available. Hues should be chosen which are neither too bland (tan) nor too bright (red). Children seem to respond well to combinations of yellow, orange, and green; adolescents prefer accents using deeper colors such as chocolate, turquoise, pumpkin, burgundy, and natural woods. Soft whites may be combined carefully in many schemes.

Wall decorations should be nonthreatening to ill children (e.g., avoid wild animals). Even favorite characters when drawn too large intimidate small children who are not feeling well. Good art, attractively mounted, may be used successfully in ambulatory settings.

Noise levels may be modified by the use of ceiling tile, carpeting, and sound-absorbent fabrics. Background noise, especially that from a television, sets up an escalating pattern: people are required to speak louder to be heard, the television volume then is increased, and voices become still louder. In contrast, a large, floor-standing aquarium that can be viewed from all sides provides a dynamic, widely appealing object of interest as well as an attractive screening device between seating zones.

Specific

Estimated space requirements (based on the inside dimensions of rooms, or net square feet) are as follows:

1. One sq ft of overall space per 3.4 annual visits.

2. Waiting room: 12 to 15 sq ft of space per seat. If a playroom is included, 20 sq ft per seat. Additional space must be allotted for toilets, telephone booths, vending machines, and so forth.

3. Reception and clerical areas: 80 sq ft per person assigned to the area, plus additional space for equipment (copy machines, computer terminals, file cabinets, and so forth).

4. Examining rooms: preferably 100 sq ft each, depending

on the amount of floor-standing equipment utilized (e.g., sphygmomanometers, suction machines), carts or tables, cupboards and shelves, sink, and the number of persons expected to occupy the room at one time (patient, parents, physician, house staff, medical students, nurse, and so forth). Estimation of total examining room space: 1 sq ft per 1.7 annual patient visits. The formula for the number of rooms required is

$$\text{(divided by)} \quad \frac{0.8 \text{ x number of annual visits x duration of visit (hours)}}{\begin{array}{c}\text{Hours per day} \\ \text{utilized}\end{array} \text{ x } \begin{array}{c}\text{number of days of} \\ \text{operation per year}\end{array}}$$

The usual allocation for a general medical patient population is two patients per examining room per hour. Examining room doorways must be wide enough to allow passage of stretchers, wheelchairs, and portable radiologic equipment. Each room should contain a sink. Suction and oxygen outlets are desirable.

5. Treatment rooms: one room, 150 sq ft, per each 10 examination rooms.

6. Utility rooms for the area are calculated on the basis of the type of supply system (central or local) and on an efficient materials management system which provides an adequate but not excessive store of essential materials: one storage room—120 to 150 sq ft; one soiled utility room—80 to 100 sq ft.

7. Offices: depending on the size of the unit, offices of 80 to 150 sq ft each may be required for the director, head nurse, social worker, and other physicians or house staff (optional).

8. A conference room with one-way mirror overlooking adjacent examining room: 300 sq ft (depends on individual need).

9. Weight, measurement, and screening room (optional): 120 sq ft.

10. Space for walls, corridors, and mechanical systems are estimated by a net-to-gross conversion factor. This factor ranges from 1.40 to 1.55 x the space required for areas 2 through 9, depending on the design of the clinic (e.g., separate staff entrance from patient space by use of multiple corridors).

11. A children's toilet and sink should be provided.

These estimates represent average space requirements and are usually modified according to architectural design and scope of professional services. Although clinic design should be flexible to allow for future expansion, movable partitions are not recommended. They must be moved 3.5 times to be cost effective, and experience indicates that partitions rarely are moved more than one time.

To be cost effective, clinic services should be planned and appointments scheduled to utilize all rooms continuously. Space may be conserved by maximum sharing of rooms by various services (e.g., general medical clinics with certain subspecialty clinics).

Basic Equipment

The following supplies and equipment should be available in the ambulatory service.

Supplies

Emesis basins
Urine collectors
Scales, infant and child
Syringes and needles, various sizes, including 21 and 23 gauge butterfly type
Collecting tubes with and without additive, including lead-free tubes
Tourniquets
Culture media, bacteriologic and fungal
Gloves, disposable
Sodium phosphate and mineral oil enema units
Refrigerator with freezing compartment
Vaccines: D-T-P, D-T, adult D-T, MMR, OPV
Tape, bandages, and gauze
Cotton balls
Alcohol sponges
Radiology illuminators

Patient file cabinets

Cotton swabs and tongue blades of various sizes

Pediatric surgical instruments including scissors, forceps, probes, curettes, and needle holders. Sutures, nylon and absorbable, gauges 2-0 to 5-0

Resuscitation cart with emergency drugs, airways, ventilation bags, and so forth

Diagnostic Equipment

Ophthalmoscope-otoscopes (may be wall mounted)

Vision tester or illuminated Snellen charts

Impedance tympanometer (may include acoustic reflex)

Screening audiometer

Sphygmomanometer with pediatric cuffs (Doppler type for infants)

Wright peak flow meter

Ultraviolet diagnostic light

Electrocardiographic equipment (may be available from cardiology services)

Refractometer, Goldberg

Microcapillary centrifuge and reader

Microscope and light

Tuberculin testing solution (PPD)

Audiovisual Equipment (for units with educational programs)

Blackboard

Projector and screen

Bulletin boards

Dental

A dentist's chair

Administration

The director of pediatric ambulatory services is in charge of all pediatric outpatient services, including the general medical clinic, and is accountable for formulating and implementing ambulatory clinic policies. If the patient volume is large, the director may delegate supervision of the medical clinic to a Board-certified pediatrician.

Records

Ambulatory pediatric medical records should be organized and maintained as recommended by the Committee on Practice and Ambulatory Medicine.[1] The director of the clinics should review the records periodically (at least monthly) to monitor the quality of care. In many settings, daily record review is necessary for quality control and teaching purposes. If the volume is large, record review may be limited to randomly selected charts. Review should include charts of subspecialty and of surgical clinics to ensure uniform quality and comprehensiveness of ambulatory care.

The clinic director or the subspecialty attending physician should review the charts of patients who fail to keep appointments. For medicolegal as well as medical reasons, an effort should be made to contact these patients to determine their progress or to arrange for another appointment.

When patients move to another geographic area, all pertinent information should be transferred or sent to their new health care providers on request. Children with chronic disorders (e.g., diabetes, asthma, sickle cell anemia, or cystic fibrosis) should carry a copy of this information with them and present it to the new physician. Transfer of information forms[1] serve the following purposes:

1. They provide a systematic method of recording all pertinent information to allow continuity of care, especially for the patient with chronic problems.

2. They enable the physician to delegate the responsibility to record pertinent data to his office and health personnel.

3. They facilitate rapid scrutiny by those concerned about the omission of routine care and important past history of both resolved and unresolved problems. They may guide the physician to update health care and to consider new avenues of investigation for continuing problems. As an alternative, a summary of a problem-oriented record may be sent.[1]

Photocopies of pertinent data (e.g., consultation, discharge summaries, and radiologic or laboratory data) should be appended. In most instances, a letter of referral will not be needed if the standard form is complete. It is inappropriate to photocopy a voluminous record or one that is illegible. For medicolegal reasons, the original record must be retained by the clinic.

The physician supervising the general medical clinic or a pediatric nurse practitioner is responsible for seeing that timely reports regarding patients are sent to referring physicians, either in private practice or on other hospital services, and to community agencies.

In urgent situations, the initial report may be telephoned. However, all verbal communications should be followed by a written report to be included in the patient's clinic record. The report should include

1. Diagnosis or problem list.

2. Pertinent laboratory or radiographic results.

3. New information elicited on history or physical examination.

4. Recommendations for therapy, follow-up, or further consultation.

5. A clear statement regarding who shall render primary care and who shall render specialized care to each patient.

To the parents of a patient, the report should include

1. Diagnosis (an explanation in lay language may be appended).

2. Recommendation for treatment and follow-up care, consultation, and preventive care.

3. Prognosis.

4. The name of the professional person directly responsible for the child's care, and alternative resources for care when that person is not available.

Quality Assurance

An accreditable clinic maintains an actively organized, peer-based quality assurance program to improve the standard of care and to promote more effective and efficient utilization of facilities and services. The organization's quality assurance program has the following characteristics:

1. Peer review of all professional and technical activities.

2. Assessment of the cost of care.

3. Review of care conducted by subunits within the organization (such as individual services, specialties, or professionals) in response to patient concerns.

4. Specific recommendations regarding appropriate, continuing education activities, changes in the organization and administration of health care delivery, or other procedures appropriate to correct the general deficiencies identified by the study.[4]

5. Follow-up to ensure that recommended actions were adequately addressed or implemented in a reasonable period of time.

6. Periodic reporting of a summary of quality assurance activities to the governing body of the organization to assist that body in meeting its responsibility to the public.

Multidisciplinary (Chronic Care) Clinic

Objectives

The chronic care clinic should be designed to provide optimal pediatric care to children who otherwise would not have such care: children who are disadvantaged physically, emotionally, neurologically, or socially. The usual specialty categorical disease clinics are not part of this concept. The objectives are to

1. Create an attitude in which each child is considered a person with a handicap rather than a handicapped child.

2. Assure each child the services of a primary pediatrician.

3. Provide access to sophisticated and coordinated pediatric medical, surgical, dental, and social care.

4. Provide a preventive or educational service during each clinic visit.

5. Facilitate each child's emotional, intellectual, social, and physical growth and development.

6. Provide each child with periodic health assessments, maintenance programs, and anticipatory guidance.

7. Provide progressive help in self care.

8. Provide access to fully inclusive and appropriate community services.

9. Develop subspecialty consultative services as required.

10. Operate on a cost-effective budget.

Clinic Design

Patients in chronic care clinics require many special services. Some of the more common areas (for a caseload of 10,000 annual patient visits) for special referral consultations include:

- nutrition: 500;
- physical medicine: 200;
- orthopedics: 300;
- neurology: 100 (may be considerably higher);
- high-risk neonate follow-up: 250;
- facial/dental: 200;
- speech and language: 1,000;
- hearing: 1,000;
- child abuse and neglect team: 50 or more.

Close affiliation should be maintained with community residential care centers for the mentally retarded and neurologically damaged, schools for the handicapped, day care stimulation centers, camps for children with multiple handicaps, community programs such as the Scouts for the handicapped, and multiple church and social agencies.

Clinic Personnel

Full-time

Chronic care clinics require a high physician/patient ratio because of the complex course of most handicapping illnesses. A minimal ratio of one pediatrician per each 5,000 annual visits is suggested. Full-time physicians should be Board-certified in pediatrics and competent in general pediatrics, ambulatory pediatrics, growth and development, care of the handicapped, community pediatrics, and leadership and management.

The high ratio also applies to the nursing staff. A nurse functioning as a primary care provider may carry a case load of up to 50 families.

Other professional personnel required to provide comprehensive services include pediatric nurse practitioners; nutritionist; audiologist; lay administrator, preferably with a background in family community health; play therapist; speech therapist; social worker.

Part-time

To supplement the function of the full-time staff and to provide consultation for complicated problems, the following professionals are required: general pediatricians, neurologist, psychiatrist, pediatric surgeon or pediatrically oriented general surgeon, pediatric dental surgeon, pediatric dentist, ambulatory pediatric fellows, otolaryngologist, orthopedic surgeon, pediatric plastic surgeon, resource person in parenting.

Estimated Space

Space requirements for services to chronically ill children usually are greater than those of a general medical clinic (see page 131). The following areas represent an ideal design for the complex services necessary, based on a patient load of 10,000 visits annually:

1. Reception area.
2. Waiting and play areas.
3. Examining rooms: 12 large and 6 small.
4. Conference areas: one large conference room, one small conference room, one nutrition conference room and office, hospital conference room or auditorium to accommodate large classes or educational meetings (may be located in another hospital area).
5. Work spaces: one nurse work room, one supply room, one reception area, one secretary and file area, six offices for professional staff.
6. Audiology room.
7. Toilets: three small, two large.
8. Screening rooms for hearing, vision, physical measurements.

Equipment

The basic equipment is that required in a general ambulatory care clinic (see pages 133-138). In addition, the following equipment is commonly available for comprehensive care:

1. Toys for Child Life Program[2]: punching bag, parallel ladder crawling toy, and play stethoscopes and otoscopes.
2. Audiology equipment: one and one-half channel audiometer for use with earphone and two speakers in soundfield.
3. Orthopedic: special wheel chairs, stretchers, crutches, casting material, and splints (*note*: sinks must contain a plaster trap).
4. Optional equipment: one closed circuit TV viewer, and one videocassette player.

Subspecialty Clinics

High quality pediatric care often involves interaction between the subspecialty consultant and the primary pediatrician. The quality of care of a growing and developing child is limited by a narrow organ-oriented approach; therefore, the following guidelines are suggested for the health supervision of a child referred for subspecialty care.

General Principles

1. Medical care in all subspecialty clinics should be coordinated by a physician with training in both the subspecialty and general pediatrics. All other clinic personnel should be trained in pediatric procedures and practice.

2. One professional person should be assigned continuing responsibility for the care and counseling of each patient and family.

3. Each clinic should provide for 24-hour and 7-day emergency coverage related to the care provided. The patient and parent should be aware of this coverage.

4. The patient's primary pediatrician or other primary health care source should receive prompt reports of all care rendered and should be consulted regarding major medical decisions. Patients without a primary physician should be referred to a source of primary care and should, when necessary, be assisted in arranging appointments.

5. Generally, subspecialty clinics are not appropriate sources of primary care. If a clinic becomes the primary source of care—and therefore the "medical home" for the patient—the clinic is responsible for a comprehensive plan for his or her care. This plan should include care of acute illness, preventive and continuing care, total health assessment, developmental assessment, appropriate screening tests and laboratory procedures, periodic reexamination, immunization, counseling, anticipatory guidance, and coordination of other care.

6. The quality of medical care received from several sources depends on the efficiency of communication. Fragmentation and duplication of care occurs when professionals fail to communicate.

Facilities and Personnel

Space and personnel needs in the pediatric subspecialties are dictated by such variables as

1. Existence of and scope of teaching program: (a) involvement of under- and postgraduate students, house staff, and fellows, and (b) associated teaching responsibilities of staff members in allied institutions.

2. Scope of research program.

3. The case load of the subspecialty services. This depends on the size and socioeconomic status of the population served and referral pattern of primary care providers in the community.

4. Cross-specialty access to services readily available (e.g., internal medicine, gynecology and obstetrics, and surgical subspecialties).

5. Access to pediatric inpatient care and ancillary services attuned to the unique needs of children, such as radiology, laboratory, child life program, and multispecialty services.

Communication

1. Improved understanding and a sense of involvement may be achieved when, in appropriate cases, the family or the patient receives a copy of the written communication, or listens to verbal communication between professionals.

2. Interpretation of the evaluation and therapy to the patient and his or her family is a responsibility shared by the referring physician and the consultant. To avoid confusion, they should agree in advance on how this interpretation is to be done.

3. When requesting subspecialty care, the referring physician should provide a clinical report by phone, letter, or mutually acceptable referral forms. Written reports have the advantage of precision and availability for later reference.

4. When reporting to the referring physician, the consultant documents: (a) additional relevant facts regarding the diagnosis(es) or general health of the patient; (b) a summary of the evaluation completed and the therapy anticipated; (c) a

plan for further evaluation and therapy, including frequency of patient visits, long-range goals, immediate objectives, and the time anticipated for their achievement; (d) an indication of the date of the next progress appraisal and report; and (e) subsequent reports to the referring physician, made regularly, to review progress toward achieving goals and objectives and to update the plan for evaluation and therapy.

References

1. Committee on Practice and Ambulatory Medicine: Management of Pediatric Practice. Elk Grove Village, Illinois: Chapter 8, in press.
2. Olds, A.R.: *In* Gellert, E., ed.: Psycho-Social Aspects of Pediatric Care. Psychological Considerations in Humanizing Physical Environment of Pediatric Outpatient and Hospital Settings. New York: Grune and Stratton, Inc., 1978.
3. For details of architectural design see Proceedings of the Symposium on Pediatric Clinic and Emergency Architecture, American Academy of Pediatrics, Section on Community Pediatrics, May, 1982.
4. Standards for Education in Ambulatory Pediatrics, Ambulatory Pediatric Association, Publication January 1, 1978.

Bibliography

Kovner, A.R., and Neuhauser, D., ed.: Health Services Management: A Book of Cases. Ann Arbor, Michigan: AUPHA Press, 1981.

Kovner, A.R., and Neuhauser, D., ed.: Health Services Management: Readings and Commentary, ed. 2. Ann Arbor, Michigan: Health Administration Press, 1983.

Rakich, J.S., and Darr, K., ed.: Hospital Organizations and Management: Text and Readings, ed. 3. New York: SP Medical & Scientific Books, 1983.

Rakich, J.S., Longest, B.B., Jr., and O'Donovan, T.R.: Managing Health Care Organizations. Hinsdale, Illinois: Dryden Press, 1977.

Rowland, H.S., and Rowland, B.L.: Hospital Administration Handbook. Rockville, Maryland: Aspen Systems Corp., 1983.

Schulz, R., and Johnson, A.C.: Management of Hospitals, ed. 2. New York: McGraw-Hill Book Co., 1983.

Chapter 14

EMERGENCY SERVICES

Emergency departments must provide a wide range of medical and surgical care for major and minor conditions. Emergency departments also should provide a 24-hour source of prompt evaluation and initial emergency stabilization for acutely ill or injured children.[1] Private primary care physicians and hospital-based emergency physicians should work together in the best interests of the patient. Interpersonal communication should be fostered so, in a crisis situation, there is no impediment to the primary care provider seeking consultation from the emergency or critical care specialist. The emergency or critical care specialist must assure timely transfer of vital patient information to the primary care provider, according to preestablished protocols, after the patient has been evaluated or treated. The capability to provide basic pediatric resuscitation and advanced pediatric life support must be continuously present in every hospital providing pediatric emergency medical care.[2]

Depending on an individual hospital's capabilities to provide pediatric emergency care, a communication system should be developed for directing pediatric patients with life-threatening conditions to the appropriate hospital. If implementation of this system reveals a potential need to transfer certain patients, the initial receiving hospital should have appropriate equipment and appropriately trained staff for initial evaluation and stabilization of pediatric patients. There should be defined transfer agreements among receiving and referral hospitals concerning the pediatric patient with life-threatening conditions.

Hospitals that do not have comprehensive pediatric inpatient services should not propose to offer comprehensive pediatric emergency care.

Hospital pediatric emergency services should be integrated into a community-based emergency plan involving all hospitals in the community which offer emergency medical services. From this community planning, emergency service resources may be classified, depending on overall capability of the hospital and medical staff to meet the needs of pediatric patients.[1]

The hospital emergency services should be coordinated with internal and external disaster plans consistent with the capabilities of the hospital and community served.[2] A communication system that permits immediate contact between hospital emergency services is needed for provision of advanced information concerning critically ill or injured patients.[2]

Close liaison with other community health care providers is essential. Every effort should be made to use an episodic illness to provide entry into a primary, continuous health care situation. A close working relationship with the public health and the human services departments is essential for appropriate follow-up of many identified health problems such as contagious disease, neglect and abuse, and social aspects of disease.

The emergency department also should serve as a resource for physician education and the education of emergency personnel; this may be done by formal training programs or by supervised clinical experience.

Categorization

The purpose of categorization of emergency medical facilities is to characterize their capability to cope with specific injuries and illnesses. If a community has more than one hospital with an emergency department, advanced knowledge of capabilities enables emergency transport systems, police, and physicians to select the appropriate hospital for each emergency.

The Commission on Emergency Medical Services of the American Medical Association formulated *Provisional Guidelines for the Optimal Categorization of Hospital Emergency Capabilities*[3] in June 1981 to help identify appropriate emergency facilities to which patients should be sent. All categories of hospital emergency facilities should offer the capability to provide basic resuscitation and advanced life support. The education and training of emergency department personnel are essential components in classification of emergency capabilities.[3]

Level I—... shall serve as a referral center for severely injured or critically ill children and for emergent diagnostic problems at any hour of the day. It should serve as an educational center in emergency and general pediatrics at all professional levels.

A physically separate pediatric emergency area is essential. There should be a full-time director of pediatric emergency care. Experienced pediatricians should be on-call and promptly available in the emergency department. Pediatric subspecialists should be on-call and promptly available.

Level II—... shall be capable of providing immediate resuscitation and life support to all pediatric patients, including newborns, as well as definitive care for most acute surgical and medical problems. A separate pediatric area of the emergency department is desirable. The staff should include a full-time emergency department director with qualified pediatricians and pediatric subspecialists on-call and promptly available. Nursing personnel with extensive training in pediatrics should be in the pediatric area at all times.

Level III—... will normally be a rural or small urban general hospital. It will appropriately treat minor illnesses and trauma and provide resuscitation and initial stabilization of seriously ill or injured patients, with referral of critically ill or injured children to higher classified facilities after stabilization.[4]

The Joint Commission on Accreditation of Hospitals categorized emergency services* in the 1984 manual as follows:

Level I—... offers comprehensive emergency care 24 hours a day, with at least one physician experienced in emergency care on duty in the emergency care area. There shall be in-hospital physician coverage by members of the medical staff or by senior-level residents for at least medical, surgical, orthopedic, obstetrical/gynecological, pediatric, and anesthesiology services. When such coverage can be demonstrated to be met suitably through another mechanism, an equivalency shall be considered to exist for purposes of compliance with the requirement. Other specialty consultation shall be available within approximately 30 minutes. Initial consultation through two-way voice communication is acceptable. The hospital's scope of services shall include in-house capabilities for managing physical and related emotional problems on a definitive basis. The above requirements also apply to a comprehensive-level emergency department/service provided by a hospital offering care only to a limited group of patients, such as pediatric, obstetrical, ophthalmological, and orthopedic.

Level II—... offers emergency care 24 hours a day, with at least one physician experienced in emergency care on duty in the emergency care

---

*Note: The sequence of levels for emergency departments is the reverse of that for neonatal intensive care units. In the latter, Level III is the most sophisticated designation.

area, and with specialty consultation available within approximately 30 minutes by members of the medical staff or by senior-level residents. Initial consultation through two-way voice communication is acceptable. The hospital's scope of services shall include in-house capabilities for managing physical and related emotional problems, with provision for patient transfer to another facility when needed.

Level III—... offers emergency care 24 hours a day, with at least one physician available to the emergency care area within approximately 30 minutes through a medical staff call roster. Initial consultation through two-way voice communication is acceptable. Specialty consultation shall be available by request of the attending medical staff member or by transfer to a designated hospital where definitive care can be provided.

Level IV—... offers reasonable care in determining whether an emergency exists, renders lifesaving first aid, and makes appropriate referral to the nearest facilities that have the capability of providing needed services. The mechanism for providing physician coverage at all times shall be defined by the medical staff.[1]

The Commission on Emergency Medical Services of the American Medical Association, the Joint Commission on Accreditation of Hospitals, and the Section on Pediatric Emergency Medicine all require that a Level I emergency department/service offer comprehensive emergency care 24 hours a day, with at least one physician experienced in emergency care on duty in the emergency care area. Consistent with this recommendation, optimal care of the pediatric victim of a critical illness or injury requires care by a career-oriented specialist in pediatric emergency medicine who devotes a majority of his or her professional time to the care of children. Other individuals involved in the delivery of pediatric emergency medical care, such as nursing and paramedical personnel, optimally also should spend a majority of their professional time in the care of children.

Physical Facilities

The physical requirements of general emergency departments have been specified by the Committee on Trauma of the American College of Surgeons.[5] These standards suffice for small hospitals. However, large general hospitals should modify the plan to make a separate children's emergency area available, with signs clearly directing pediatric patients and their families to this area.

The emergency area should be located on a ground floor to facilitate the transfer of patients from the entrance to the treatment area. Pediatric emergency facilities should be clearly marked and delineated. Ramps are necessary for wheelchairs and stretchers if there are any steps or other elevations.

The physicians' and nurses' station area should have maximum visibility of the emergency department. Copies of the hospital's and emergency department's operating policies and procedures should be kept in a central station area for ready reference. A bulletin board is essential for transmitting current information to personnel and maintaining rosters of personnel on call. A magnetic board with color-coded magnets for posting patient information is an invaluable aid for managing a busy emergency department.

Parking should be adjacent to the emergency entrance and adequately controlled to ensure space for patients and staff at all times. There also should be sufficient space at the emergency entrance door to unload patients; this area should be covered or enclosed to protect patients from the elements during transfer from the ambulance or car. The pedestrian entrance and the ambulance entrance should be separated to avoid interference with immediate admission of critically ill or injured children. This separation also protects those waiting from additional distress by observing the critically ill or injured patients.

Wheelchair and stretcher storage space should be provided at the entrance; the stretcher should have adjustable side rails and adequate restraints. A heated incubator or warmer for high-risk infants should be immediately available at the emergency entrance.

The pediatric emergency department should be adjacent to at least one elevator limited to the transfer of patients and professional personnel to the operating rooms, intensive care units, and other hospital areas.

A well defined pediatric subunit should be identified in the emergency department of large general hospitals, and all children should be triaged immediately to this area. If space is available, a subunit should include a separate pediatric waiting room.

Large emergency departments, especially referral centers, may have a heliport adjacent to, but at a safe distance from, the entrance. A landing area approximately 100 ft x 100 ft is required. There should be two lines of approach or take-off which are removed from each other by at least a 90 degree angle and free of obstructions when in a path computed on a ratio of 8 ft horizontal to 1 ft vertical. Local government agencies may have additional legal requirements. The landing area must be clearly marked to be readily visible from the air, and it must be well lighted at night. A minimum of 120 BC size, dry powder fire extinguisher must be available at the helicopter site.

Functional Organization

Space requirements of pediatric emergency units frequently are underestimated, resulting in small and inefficient cubicles. The small size of a child's body is unrelated to the space required for care. Because one to four persons usually accompany each pediatric patient, seating must be available for parents and siblings in the waiting room and sometimes in the examination rooms. The total space requirement of a pediatric emergency department is 0.1 to 0.2 sq ft of space per annual pediatric emergency department patient visit. The number of treatment rooms may be estimated based on the formula of 2,000 annual visits per treatment room. By multiplying the total number of treatment rooms by 620 gross sq ft, the total space requirements for the entire emergency department can be projected. Another method for determining space needed utilizes a formula of 6.60 visits per gross sq ft, which equates to 25,000 visits per 3,600 gross sq ft. Estimates of area, based on "rules of thumb," must not be used for anything more than a crude reference.[6]

A large pediatric emergency department may be organized into distinct functional units, which include:
1. Triage.
2. Registration/waiting.
3. Trauma/critical.
4. Observation/holding.
5. Examination/ambulatory.
6. Discharge/collections.
7. Ancillary support.

8. Other: (a) patient conference room, (b) patient/staff education conference room, (c) poison control center, (d) physician on-call/locker rooms, (e) staff offices.

The basic operating assumption of the design and construction of individual examining rooms is that patients who are in emergency departments, regardless of their triage category, are potentially life threatened. This requires that every treatment and every examining room be designed to allow appropriate lifesaving procedures to be carried out. Every room within the emergency department should include oxygen and suction mounted on the wall. An adequate number of electrical outlets must be available for the equipment required if a resuscitation becomes necessary. The doorways should open wide enough to allow a second cart to be wheeled in if the patient requires transport to a resuscitation suite or another part of the hospital. Communication equipment should be available, i.e., an intercom in each room to allow for help to be rapidly summoned to any part of the emergency department. All electrical and other outlets should be childproofed to prevent secondary injury while the child is in the room.[7]

The design of the department should carefully balance the genuine medical need for close patient observation and immediate communication with the equally important patient need for privacy. There is a sensitive balance between intrusion of privacy and isolation/abandonment.[8] Achieving this balance depends on having a staff commitment to emergency evaluation, treatment, and total care of the family.

Triage Area

Pediatric patients in the emergency department should be assessed on arrival to determine if they require urgent treatment. The triage unit is a specifically designated area which should be adjacent to the entrance. It should be staffed by experienced personnel whose primary function is to assess the degree of medical urgency and direct the patient to the appropriate channel of service.

Triage may be performed by an experienced physician, such

as a senior pediatric resident, or by a specially trained nurse or pediatric nurse associate. The triage person should be capable of making quick, accurate judgments and relate well to the patient's and caretaker's concerns. However, first aid measures should not be performed in triage. The triage person may use the following guidelines to categorize patients.

Priority I: Emergency (Color Coded Red)

Pediatric patients whose condition is life threatening or will cause serious, permanent, physical impairment if not treated immediately (e.g., convulsions, hemorrhage, severe burns, shock, severe trauma, epiglottitis, respiratory or cardiopulmonary arrest) should be referred immediately to the trauma/critical care area.

Priority II: Urgent (Color Coded Yellow)

The condition of patients who require care within 30 minutes to 2 hours would not generally cause loss of life or serious, permanent impairment if treatment is deferred (e.g., moderate burns, hyperpyrexia, mild croup, dislocations). They should be referred to the examination/ambulatory care area for prompt evaluation.

Priority III: Nonurgent (Color Coded Green)

Speed of evaluation is not critical for patients whose condition is not serious (e.g., abrasion, nasal or mild pharyngeal congestion, insect bites with local reaction, conjunctivitis). However, they should be evaluated as soon as possible. This determination should be made only by experienced physicians after sufficient examination of the patient. Particular care is needed for neonates and infants.

Management in the Triage Area

Psychiatric disorders of childhood may fall into any category and require particular sensitivity by the triage person.

Whenever the patient, caretaker, and accompanying interested members of the "extended family" are required to wait until the patient can be examined by the physician, they should be made comfortable. Sensitivity to their emotional and physical needs by members of the hospital staff is an essential component of pediatric emergency care.

Chronic minor complaints and complex chronic illnesses or behavior problems may be seen last or referred elsewhere. These patients should be given assurance that the condition is not urgent and assisted in obtaining an appointment to another facility.

High-risk newborn infants accompanied by a physician-directed transport team should be transferred directly to the neonatal intensive care unit. An effective communication system from the ambulance to the emergency department will allow for expeditious handling of this type of transfer. However, newborn infants born out of a hospital and those referred from surrounding hospitals and sent by conventional ambulance should be evaluated immediately on arrival. There should be specialized equipment and trained staff in the department for emergency resuscitation of newborn infants.

Registration/Waiting Area

Just as the street approach to the emergency department must be clearly defined by illuminated signs, the registration area should be clearly identified. The traffic must flow without interference from entry to triage and directly from triage to either the registration or the critical care area.

The registration area should be an inviting facility where people are able to sit down while filling out forms or giving necessary information. The patient and companion should feel that they are more important than paper work.[8] Attention to seating arrangements, colors, acoustics, lighting, and reading materials are a few of the many important factors influencing the perception of stress during registration and waiting. The size of the waiting area should be determined by allowing 20 sq ft of space per maximum patient occupancy. An adjacent playroom is recommended, but it must be supervised. Waiting facilities should include toilets, a drinking fountain, and public telephones. Receptionists should be pleasant and interested in the patients' and parents' comfort and welfare.

The registration process should not be time consuming. Use of computers, including key punch and visual display, can shorten the registration process and generate a patient chart within 10 minutes.

The registration information includes patient's name; date and time of arrival; patient identification number; birth date and age; sex; race; name of parent, guardian, or responsible party; current address and telephone number if they are different from that of the patient; name of the primary care provider; and type of financial coverage. There also must be a place for the signature of the responsible party giving informed consent for treatment (in the appropriate language). If the patient is critically ill or injured, the patient's condition always must take priority over completion of registration forms.

Trauma/Critical Care Area

The trauma and critical care areas of the emergency department must be capable of providing advanced pediatric life support immediately at any moment, 24 hours a day, to a pediatric victim of a critical illness or injury regardless of the patient's size. This requires specialized design incorporating the following:

1. From 220 to 240 sq ft (however, the upper limit may range as high as 350 sq ft per bed) of space per stretcher.

2. Wall-mounted oxygen, air, and suction.

3. Multiple, grounded electrical outlets.

4. Capability for continuous cardiac and respiratory monitoring/defibrillation.

5. Infusion controller/pump.

6. Capability for maintaining neutral thermal environment for exposed patients (warmer or lamps).

7. Wall-mounted pegboard with labeled essential equipment/supplies.

8. Wall-mounted patient condition board for recording serial observations and medications/treatments given.

9. Adequate room size for full cardiopulmonary resuscitation team attendance.

10. Chart with essential medications and dosages prominently displayed.

The ratio of trauma and critical care areas to total patient care areas should be appropriate for the ratio of critical to total patients for an individual facility; however, at least one treatment room should be designed, equipped, and designated for this purpose.

Observation and Holding Areas

Observation and holding areas are an essential component of the emergency department. Patients may be held for observation and treatment for several hours pending a decision on whether they can be released safely or require hospital admission. However, written guidelines defining eligible conditions, appropriate therapy, length of stay in the unit, and responsibility for determination of discharge or admission should be documented. The area should be equipped with appropriate monitors for providing cardiopulmonary resuscitation; however, it is not recommended that the observation area be used for or replace the intensive care unit. Depending on the spatial relationships within the emergency department, separate nurse staffing may be necessary. Children who require extensive monitoring should be transferred to the intensive care unit as soon as possible.

Examination and Ambulatory Care Areas

The examination and ambulatory care areas are designed for the care of minor surgical problems and acute illnesses.

Because several people generally accompany a pediatric emergency department patient and are present during the examination, the examination room should be 100 to 120 sq ft.[9] Furnishings should include plastic, cleanable chairs for parents and the physician; adjustable examination tables; an instrument table or counter; and a covered waste container. An alarm, bell button, or signal light switch should be installed within arm's length of the examining table in every treatment room. There should be intercom communication to the central nursing desk. One unit should have a chair and equipment suitable for eye, ear, nose, throat, or dental examinations. Wall suction and oxygen are assets in examination rooms, and suction and compressed air are essential in rooms used for eye, ear, nose, and throat examinations. One unit should have a table with stirrups and appropriate lighting for genitalia and pelvic examinations. Each room should be equipped with a sink for proper hand washing. A plaster trap must be incorporated into the sinks in the rooms used for plaster application.

Discharge and Collection Areas

Planning must be made for an appropriate area to carry out discharge instructions and follow-up plans. There must be documentation that the responsible party understands the discharge instructions and a follow-up plan emphasizing continuity of care. If the emergency department serves foreign-speaking populations, it may be necessary to staff the emergency department with bilingual personnel and print educational materials and discharge instructions in more than one language.

The financial billing and collection area should assign definite accountability for financial settlement for services rendered in an environment of privacy and comfort. Although emergency care must not be predicated on the ability to pay, those who repeatedly misuse the emergency department for nonemergency conditions may be counseled at the time of discharge (after care is given) concerning alternative providers of nonemergency care in the community.

Ancillary Support Areas

It may be necessary to incorporate a satellite laboratory or satellite radiographic room within the emergency department, depending on the volume of tests needed and the location of the emergency department in relation to those areas in the main hospital. Immediate return of critical laboratory tests and radiographs may necessitate the proximity provided by satellite services.

Other

Many other special areas are needed in the emergency department, including adequate rest rooms with tables for diaper changing, poison information center, patient/parent conference room (e.g., interview, isolation, grieving), staff education/conference room, staff offices, on-call room, locker rooms, utility rooms, major equipment storage rooms, and a central nursing area with ice machine, refrigerators, and medications.

Note: The more pediatric patients an emergency department treats, the more necessary it becomes to have immediate access to comprehensive poison information systems.

Administrative Organization

Pediatric emergency department policies should be formulated by the director of the department, the chief of staff or pediatric department chairman, the nursing supervisor, the administrator, and a committee representing the various disciplines. There is a growing trend in large general hospitals to staff emergency departments with full-time, career-oriented specialists in emergency medicine. If there is an adequate annual volume of pediatric patients, they should be separated from adult patients and seen by specialists in pediatric emergency medicine who spend the majority of their professional time in the care of children. Standards of care for all infants and children, regardless of where the care is rendered in the hospital, should be primarily the responsibility of the pediatric staff.

One function of the emergency department director is to recruit qualified pediatric emergency department professional personnel, with the advice and cooperation of the directors of nursing, social services, and surgery. The director also should establish liaison with other departments in the hospital and with practitioners in the community to ensure prompt care of referred patients.

Training and supervision in emergency diagnosis, cardiopulmonary resuscitation, and the appropriate use of laboratory and radiology services should be provided for the house staff in the emergency department. An emergency department manual should be formulated for standard rules and procedures, and a plan should be established for disaster situations. Patient records should be reviewed routinely; based on this review, emergency care should be upgraded. Training courses in resuscitation and emergency care should be organized for physician's assistants, ambulance attendants, firemen, policemen, and other appropriate members of the community. To mitigate the stressful effects of continuous employment in the emergency room, stress management sessions for staff should be considered.

Relationships of the emergency department to other departments within the hospital, as well as relationships of the director of emergency services with other members of the medical staff, should be defined.[2]

An emergency division administrator responsible to the director is desirable. The administrator's duties include (1) hiring and supervision of allied health and secretarial personnel; (2) ordering and maintaining equipment and supplies; (3) supervision of housekeeping within a department; (4) establishing liaison with community agencies; (5) recording and analyzing data relating to cost, patient volume, laboratory utilization, and so forth; and (6) any other administrative duties assigned by the director.

Personnel

Nursing service personnel should be accountable primarily to the director of the pediatric emergency department. The head nurse is responsible for hiring personnel and for developing schedules and duties of all personnel, including registered nurses, licensed practical nurses, and emergency medical technicians. The head nurse should assist in the preparation of a manual of standard procedures for the department and develop a similar manual for the nursing personnel. The head nurse, in lieu of a unit administrator, also may review and order equipment and supplies.

If registered nurses are trained and experienced, their duties may include the triage of patients in receiving areas to ensure that true emergencies are handled promptly.

Physician's assistants and pediatric nurse practitioners may perform certain emergency department duties under the supervision of a physician, who assumes responsibility. These duties may include taking the history, performing a physical examination, assisting in routine laboratory and screening procedures (e.g., blood tests, urinalysis, cultures), removing sutures or casts, applying wound dressings, performing minor incision and drainage, and strapping or splinting sprains. All professional and paraprofessional personnel should be trained in basic cardiopulmonary resuscitation, and this training should be updated frequently.

Clerks and receptionists relieve professional personnel of administrative and other duties not requiring medical training (e.g., reception and registration of patients, completion of forms, telephone answering, and collections).

If consultants in various specialties (e.g., dentistry, ophthalmology, orthopedics, psychiatry) are not immediately available, a plan should be defined for transfer to a facility where they are.

The social services representative responsible to the emergency department should assist in dealing with the social and environmental problems associated with delivery of pediatric emergency care. The prime reason for many emergency visits may be social rather than medical (e.g., lack of adequate physical care, drug abuse, child neglect). A method for integrating this service into a package of total care should be developed.

Note: The reporting relationships may vary according to the internal organizational structure of the hospital.

Records

Every patient visit should be recorded permanently, and all entries should be legible. In addition to previously mentioned registration information, the emergency department record should contain the following information:

1. Triage category.

2. A concise history of illness or injury, including pertinent negative history.

3. Medications given prior to arrival.

4. A history of immunization status.

5. A history of drug allergies.

6. Complete vital signs and weight.

7. Physical examination, including pertinent negative findings.

8. Laboratory and radiologic findings.

9. Diagnosis.

10. Emergency treatment, including drug dosage and route of administration.

11. Record of consultants or contacts (police, social services) involved in delivery of care.

12. Condition at discharge.

13. Discharge disposition of the patient.

14. Signature of the examining physician.

15. Signature of the nurse responsible for carrying out treatments and discharge instructions.

16. Signature of the responsible party who documents understanding of discharge instructions regarding home care and follow-up.

17. Time of discharge.

Ideally, all charts should be dictated and, therefore, easily reviewed in duplicate, with a copy sent to the primary care provider. All complex, complicated cases, including those with a potential for court review (e.g., child abuse, sexual abuse, rape) should be dictated. All complete hospital medical records should be available for all patients being examined. A unit record system provides the best assurance that previous visits or hospitalizations will be part of the same record.

Manual of Standard Operating Procedures

A reference manual of standard procedures and policies should be available in the pediatric emergency department and include the following:

1. The objectives of delivery of emergency care.
2. The lines of administrative authority.
3. Job descriptions or clarification of professional responsibility.
4. Permissible procedures or therapy that can be carried out in the emergency department.
5. Protocol for follow-up care.
6. Procedures for utilization of the observation area.
7. Procedures for transfer of patients to other areas of the hospital or to other institutions.
8. Procedures for procuring current toxicology information (e.g., from a regional poison control center).
9. Disposition of suspected child abuse and sexual misuse/abuse cases.
10. Methods for 24-hour procurement of supplies, equipment, and drugs.
11. Specifications for medical staff coverage.
12. Communication with local health authorities and police about accidents, unexplained trauma, drug overdose, rage, contagious disease, and other reportable conditions.
13. Plans for communication by telephone and telemetry with emergency transport systems and with professional and paramedical personnel at the site.
14. Plans for handling special situations (e.g., children dead on arrival, patients or parents under the influence of drugs, emancipated minors, suspected rape or pregnancy, psychotic children or parents, and care of minors unaccompanied by a parent or legal guardian).
15. A disaster plan with provision for handling or disposition of mass casualties (the hospital's disaster plan should

be integrated with the community's disaster plan).[10]

16. Regulations pertaining to consent and exceptions.

The procedure and policy manual will require periodic revision. The emergency department director and/or responsible committee of the medical staff, with the assistance of the medical and nursing staff, is responsible for updating the manual.

Quality Control

There should be a planned program for ongoing review and evaluation of the quality and appropriateness of patient care provided in the emergency department. The physician director and/or committee of the medical staff is responsible for implementing the review and evaluation program, which should be integrated into the hospital's quality assurance program.

Through review and assessment of information obtained from ongoing monitoring activities and other data sources, important problems in patient care, and opportunities for improving care are identified. The chart of all patients leaving prior to physician evaluation and of patients dying in the emergency department should be carefully reviewed.

Appropriate action should be taken to resolve identified problems, and the effectiveness of these actions should be documented.[11]

Education

The emergency department offers an unparalleled opportunity for the education of all levels of medical personnel to develop accurate clinical judgment in the care of critically ill or injured children.

Emergency department education programs may be directed toward physicians, nurses, or allied health personnel. Outlines of training programs have been developed for advanced emergency medical technicians, physician's assistants, medical students, and house staff. The emergency department staff has responsibility for supporting educational activities throughout the entire emergency medical services network for the community. This may include provision of advanced pediatric life support training to emergency medical technicians, police and fire department personnel, school health personnel, and the emergency department staff of other hospitals. Only through a sense of responsibility to the system of emergency medical services delivery of pediatric emergency medical care can critical pediatric victims of illness and injury receive prompt and appropriate specialized care.

References

1. Accreditation Manual for Hospitals (AMH/85). Chicago: Joint Commission on Accreditation of Hospitals, p. 18, 1984.
2. Accreditation Manual for Hospitals (AMH/85). Chicago: Joint Commission on Accreditation of Hospitals, p. 19, 1984.
3. Commission on Emergency Medical Services: Provisional Guidelines for the Optimal Categorization of Hospital Emergency Capabilities. Chicago: American Medical Association, pp. 1, 4, 1982.
4. Commission on Emergency Medical Services: Provisional Guidelines for the Optimal Categorization of Hospital Emergency Capabilities. Chicago: American Medical Association, p. 29, 1982.
5. Committee on Trauma/70: Guidelines for Design and Function of a Hospital Emergency Department. Chicago: American College of Surgeons, 1970.
6. Tyne, M.: Planning for pediatric emergency and ambulatory care facilities. *In* Section on Community Pediatrics: Proceedings of the Symposium on Pediatric Clinic and Emergency Architecture, June 26-28, 1981, Chicago. Evanston, Illinois: American Academy of Pediatrics, unpublished manuscript.
7. Lumpkin, J.: Observations from the viewpoint of the emergency physician. *In* Section on Community Pediatrics: Proceedings of the Symposium on Pediatric Clinic and Emergency Architecture, June 26-28, 1981, Chicago. Evanston, Illinois: American Academy of Pediatrics, unpublished manuscript.
8. Petersen, R.: Behavioral design in OPD architecture: Consideration for reception and waiting areas. *In* Section on Community Pediatrics: Proceedings of the Symposium on Pediatric Clinic

and Emergency Architecture, June 26-28, 1981, Chicago. Evanston, Illinois: American Academy of Pediatrics, unpublished manuscript.

9. Baushard, R.B., and Gates, R.S.: Factors to be considered in the planning phase. *In* Section on Community Pediatrics: Proceedings of the Symposium on Pediatric Clinic and Emergency Architecture, June 26-28, 1981, Chicago. Evanston, Illinois: American Academy of Pediatrics, unpublished manuscript.

10. Accreditation Manual for Hospitals (AMH/85). Chicago: Joint Commission on Accreditation of Hospitals, p. 132, 1984.

11. Accreditation Manual for Hospitals (AMH/85). Chicago: Joint Commission on Accreditation of Hospitals, p. 28, 1984.

12. Subcommittee on Emergency Cardiac Care: Textbook of Advanced Cardiac Life Support. Dallas, Texas: American Heart Association, 1983.

Addendum

Pediatric Emergency Care Equipment

The following equipment must be appropriately sized to provide care to all pediatric patients from newborn infants through adolescents:

- indwelling peripheral vein catheters;
- saphenous vein cutdown;
- assorted intravenous fluids;
- arterial line (including umbilical artery);
- continuous blood pressure monitoring;
- central venous line;
- infusion controller;
- bag-valve-mask for delivery of variable oxygen concentration up to 100%;
- blood warmer*;
- endotracheal tubes and blades (orotracheal and nasotracheal equipment);
- suction and suction catheters;
- nasogastric tubes;
- pediatric mechanical ventilator;

---

*Particularly critical for care of infants or younger children.

- essential medications (see *Textbook of Advanced Cardiac Life Support*[12]);
- portable, continuous cardiac and respiratory monitoring/ defibrillator with pediatric paddles;
- equipment for tracheotomy;
- equipment for thoracotomy;
- transfusion and autotransfusion equipment;
- scales with kilogram measurements;
- lumbar puncture tray;
- mast trousers (medical antishock trousers);
- radiant warmer*;
- hypothermic thermometers*;
- transport incubator*;
- disposable tapes for measurement of head and abdominal circumference.

---

*Particularly critical for care of infants or younger children.

Chapter 15

RADIOLOGY SERVICES

The referring physician today is presented with an almost bewildering array of imaging techniques, each offering a different kind of information and level of risk. Because many of the diagnostic imaging techniques are recently developed, there is much to learn about which technique or techniques are most effective in many situations.

Roentgenograms (x-ray films) are the most frequently used diagnostic imaging technique, but they have been supplemented with other methods and techniques that use other forms of energy: radioisotopes, ultrasound, and a combination of strong magnetic fields and radiowaves. The available methods are shown in Table 4.

Each of the imaging methods, and the many procedures used with them (such as angiography and cardiac imaging), have advantages in the evaluation of certain conditions. The first two groups carry some risk because they involve ionizing radiation, and in some instances this risk is greater for pediatric patients than adults.

Most imaging procedures are performed by radiologists or nuclear medicine physicians. Hospitals with pediatric services should have at least one radiologist who is interested in children and their diseases. In many situations, the pediatrician and pediatric radiologist should consult to determine the imaging studies to be performed. This choice should depend not only on the recommendations in the medical literature but also on the availability of appropriate equipment and the experience of the medical imager(s) involved. Occasionally a child should be referred to another hospital or clinic for specific imaging procedures; few hospitals can afford all of the types of equipment and can provide the expertise required to do all types of pediatric imaging well.

Patient Care

In the imaging department(s), as on the nursing units, young patients require substantially more care and supervision than adult patients. This care should be provided by trained, reliable people who enjoy helping sick children.

Many medical imaging examinations are especially frightening to small children. The equipment is strange and often large. The child is placed in positions that frequently are uncomfortable and is told to hold still. Sandbags, adhesive tape, and special devices frequently are used to hold the child in the proper position.

Efforts should be made to make children feel at ease with the equipment. Their fears will be lessened if the imaging area suggests there are people about who will like them: cheerful cartoon and fairy tale friends on the walls and imaging machines and, if possible, a play area with carefully selected toys in the waiting room. Most important, they should be attended by at least one person who clearly cares about them (a technologist, nurse, or other trained individual in the imaging department) and who can (1) explain in words appropriate to the child's development the procedure that is about to be performed, (2) show the child the imaging machine that will be used and explain how the child will relate to that machine during the examination, (3) show the child the method that will be used to help him hold still, and (4) allay the child's fears as the examination proceeds.

Ultrasound can be explained to children easily as they can play with the equipment—creating images on the screen and erasing them—before it is used on them. With many Beta (β)-scanners, the sonographer can write the child's name in the air. The name appears on the screen, and the child can be given a polaroid picture of it. However, the child's cooperation may be lost if the mineral oil or gel spread on his or her skin is not comfortably warm.

Premature infants should be examined in the incubator or warmer whenever possible. When they must be removed, they should be kept under a warming lamp or on a warming pad, or both.

The pediatric radiologist should train a number of technologists in the special care and techniques necessary to make excellent images of children. At a minimum, the imaging department should arrange its schedule so that all examinations of children, both those done at the bedside and those done in the radiology department, are performed by the specially trained technologists on appropriate equipment. If possible, specific imaging equipment should be designated primarily for pediatric examinations.

Infants and young children usually cannot be examined as quickly as ambulatory adults. The imaging department should allot ample time to perform these studies and assign two technologists, or a technologist and another trained individual, to each examination of an infant or a young child.

Parents

Children's fears are intensified by separation from their parents. Frequently it is easier to examine a child if a parent is within the child's vision. Parents who are in the room when an x-ray exposure is made should wear a lead apron. If there is any possibility that the mother may be pregnant, she should step out of the room or behind a radiation barrier when the exposure is made.

Protection from Injury

Children must be protected from injury on their way to and from the imaging department and while there. Infants and young children never should be left unattended in the examining room. During each examination, one person should watch the child at all times and be close enough to react promptly should the child experience any difficulty. Infants and small children frequently must be immobilized for examinations. This should be done by experienced technologists who realize that all methods for immobilization present a slight hazard and know how to deal with adverse reactions.

It is difficult to watch an infant or small child under a fluoroscope, particularly when the lights are dim. With modern image intensification, there is no reason to fluoroscope in a darkened room. The light should be kept sufficiently bright so the child can be observed carefully all the time. It is even more difficult to see an infant or small child in the large gantries used for CT and NMR. In many CT and NMR examining rooms, children should be monitored with closed circuit television, physiologic monitors, or both.

Oxygen and suction should be available quickly in the examining rooms as should two emergency carts—one with equipment, drugs, and drug doses for infants and children, and one similarly equipped for adults and large adolescents.

Equipment and Techniques

In all diagnostic tests that use ionizing radiation—x-rays and radioisotopes—the guiding principle should be ALARA, "As Little As Reasonably Achievable." This is particularly important when the tests are performed on infants and children. As far as is known, diagnostic ultrasound and nuclear magnetic resonance are safe for humans. However, long-term epidemiologic studies have not been performed on children; so examinations on children should be limited to what is required for diagnosis.

In all imaging studies, the dose must not be so drastically reduced that it jeopardizes the success of the study. The physician performing or supervising each study needs to have as much information as possible about the patient's illness and the results of all diagnostic tests to date so that he or she can tailor the imaging study to yield all the required information with the smallest dose. One reason for repeat studies—and frequently with needless radiation exposure—is that the referring physician has not told the imager what he or she wishes to learn from the examination. For this reason, the form requesting imaging consultation ideally should have spaces to write (1) a summary of the history and physical findings; (2) the results of previous imaging studies, especially those performed in a separate department, hospital, or office; (3) the diagnosis or diagnoses entertained; and (4) an answer to the question, "What information do you wish to learn from this examination?" In complicated cases, the information provided on the form should be supplemented by verbal consultation.

X-rays

X-ray film and intensifying screens should be used that require as little radiation as possible for a technically excellent examination. The x-ray beam should be limited to the portion of the body to be examined. Relatively small errors in alignment of the x-ray tube or in positioning the patient are much more significant in small patients than in adults. To minimize absorbed radiation, kilovoltage should be as high as is compatible with a technically excellent study. A gonad shield should be used whenever a boy has descended testicles that are within or near the primary x-ray beam. During examinations of the lower abdomen and pelvis of girls, it seldom is possible to shield the ovaries without obscuring findings that may be the key to the diagnosis. Fortunately, in comparable examination of boys and girls of similar size, the dose absorbed by the ovaries is considerably less than the dose absorbed by the unshielded testicles.

Radioisotopes

The radioisotope dose used for a child is smaller than that for an adult. Various formulas are used to calculate the dose. In general, they are based on age, body weight, body surface area, or a combination of these factors. Differences in the biodistribution of radioisotopes in children as compared to that of adults may alter the required dose considerably. Moreover, the type of equipment available, the technique used, and the cooperation of the patient influence the dose required to achieve an adequate study. In general, most radioisotope studies today deliver the same or less radiation than x-ray studies that supply comparable information.

Ultrasound

Real-time ultrasound, using a sector scanner, is preferred for most pediatric work because the small-headed transducer can be used where access is difficult, such as between ribs; and real-time equipment allows the use of ultrasound when the child is wriggling or crying. Up to about 1½ years old, the 5 or 7 MHz sector scanner also can be used through the anterior fontanelle for brain images. Static scanners (articulated arm scanners and β-scanners) are needed only when the pathologic process is larger than the field of view of the imaging system (e.g., large Wilms' tumor or hepatoblastoma) to document the relationship of the mass to surrounding structures.

The examination of a child by ultrasound should be performed by an experienced radiologist or sonographer familiar with the handling of children. If the procedure is performed by a sonographer, the radiologist must be readily available to participate in the examination; static films often do not adequately demonstrate observations made during real-time or β-mode imaging. Even videotaping may not adequately reflect the mind-hand image coordination required to make a diagnosis.

Immobilization

One of the chief problems in obtaining satisfactory radiographic studies of infants and young children is patient motion. Immobilization methods and devices should be chosen that are efficient yet as safe and pleasant as possible. The child, of course, is not truly immobilized; motion is only limited and breathing must not be restricted. Consequently, fast exposures are important, and radiographic equipment should be chosen that allows exposures of 3 milliseconds or less (8 milliseconds for bedside equipment).

Low Efficacy Examinations

Routine Chest Roentgenograms

Screening for tuberculosis is now the province of the tuberculin test rather than the chest roentgenogram. The amount of clinically important information gained by making routine chest roentgenograms of infants, children, and adolescents on admission to the hospital or before surgery is too little to justify either the expense or the radiation exposure.[1-3] If the child has symptoms or signs suggesting chest or cardiac disease, chest roentgenograms may well be indicated. They usually should be obtained before operations on the chest, and they probably should be obtained before major surgery of the face, neck, or other sites during which aspiration into the trachea and bronchi is likely to occur.

Other Routine Imaging Examinations

It is unlikely that routine imaging examinations of children are justified.

Skull X-ray Examinations After Trauma

Studies have reported that most children with head injuries do not need x-ray examinations of the skull.[4,5] Moreover, when this type of examination is indicated, CT examination frequently is preferable to skull roentgenograms; the critical factor is whether the trauma has damaged intracranial structures. Various criteria for obtaining skull roentgenograms or CT examinations have been developed, including recently proposed criteria for children (see Table 5).[5]

Other Radiographic Examinations

Siebert and colleagues[6] critically reviewed the x-ray examinations done at their hospital and concluded that some are seldom indicated and others are indicated only in certain circumstances. Although many pediatricians and radiologists probably do not agree with all of their recommendations, they merit consideration.

Conclusion

The past decade has witnessed a dramatic increase in diagnostic imaging techniques, nearly all of which are applicable in pediatrics. Advantages of the new techniques include (1) more precise diagnosis in many areas (e.g., visualization of pancreatic pseudocysts); (2) increased patient comfort (e.g., CT brain scans versus pneumoencephalography); and (3) decreased radiation (e.g., ultrasound versus intravenous urography for hydronephrosis). Guidelines for the most accurate and expeditious way to approach diagnoses are still being established in many areas of medicine. Especially during this period, pediatricians frequently will be well advised to consult with the radiologist or other medical imager rather than merely to order an examination.

References

1. Farnsworth, P.B., Steiner, E., Klein, R.M., and San Fillippo, J.A.: The value of routine preoperative chest roentgenograms in infants and children. J.A.M.A., 244:582, 1980.
2. Neuhauser, D.: Cost-effective clinical decision making. Pediatrics, 60:756, 1977.
3. Sagel, S.S., Evens, R.G., Forrest, J.V., and Bramson, R.T.: Efficacy of routine screening and lateral chest radiographs in a hospital-based population. New Engl. J. Med., 291:1001, 1974.
4. Bell, R.S., and Loop, J.W.: The utility and futility of radiographic skull examination for trauma. New Engl. J. Med., 284:236, 1971.
5. Leonidas, J.C., Ting, W., Binkiewicz, A., Vaz, R., Scott, R.M.,

and Pauker, S.G.: Mild head trauma in children: When is a roentgenogram necessary? Pediatrics, 69:139, 1982.

6. Siebert, J.J., Bryant, E., Lowe, B.A., Fiser, R., Euler, A., Byrne, W.J., Sarnat, H.B., Jones, J., Redman, J., Morrissy, R.T., Golladay, E.S., and Siebert, R.W.: Low efficacy radiography of children. Amer. J. Roentgen., 134:1219, 1980.

Table 4

Diagnostic Imaging Techniques

X-rays (Roentgen Rays)	Radioisotopes (Nuclear Medicine)	Ultrasound	Combined Strong Magnetic Fields and Radiowaves
Static radiography Fluoroscopy with cine and videotape recording Tomography, conventional Digital x-ray imaging static radiography fluoroscopy computed (axial) tomography (CT or CAT)	Scintigraphy flow static Single photon emission computed tomography (SPECT) Position emission computed tomography (PET)	Static images α-mode scans β-mode scans Dynamic images real-time ultrasound 2-dimensional echocardi- ography	Nuclear magnetic resonance imaging (NMR)

Table 5

Criteria for Skull Examinations

Historical Criteria	Physical Examination Criteria
Age below 1 year Unconsciousness longer than 5 minutes Gunshot wound or skull penetration Previous craniotomy with shunting tube in place	Palpable hematoma on scalp Skull depression palpated or identified by probe in scalp laceration CSF discharge from ear or nose Blood in middle ear Battle sign Raccoon eyes Lethargy, coma, or stupor Focal neurologic signs

Chapter 16

DIAGNOSTIC SERVICES

General Considerations

The laboratory should be service oriented and provide a repertoire of tests, a schedule of availability, and published turn-around times commensurate with clinical need. Valid needs for relevant laboratory data used in critical care situations must be met with appropriate laboratory response. Table 6 shows a representative partial list of tests available on a "STAT" basis and response times for these test results. Response times must be determined within individual institutions according to characteristics of the local laboratory, such as staff, instrumentation, and specific technique for a given test. Exceptions to established response times can be expected when unusual circumstances affect a laboratory's operations.

Quality control and quality assurance programs should be conspicuous. Test result data should be presented in a manner which facilitates recognition of "panic values" and abnormal results based on age-related reference values. Consultation on interpretation of test results should be available.

The director of laboratories should be a Board-certified pathologist who participates in hospital governance, interdepartmental clinical care, and educational activities.

In tertiary care units, specific studies may be done in a laboratory geographically associated with the unit to improve efficiency and shorten response time.

Specimen Procurement

The pediatric patient should be treated with respect and care, and specimens should be obtained in a professional manner. The techniques for obtaining blood by skin puncture should be carried out with the child's safety foremost in mind.

"Heel sticks" should be done only by trained personnel with an understanding of the anatomy and hazards associated with infection and scarring of the plantar surface of the foot. Careful warming of the skin puncture site facilitates blood flow and "arterialization" of the sample. Specimens in excess of 1.2 ml are best procured by venipuncture; arterial puncture should be carried out only by specially trained personnel.

All specimens must be properly labeled and accompanied by a properly executed request for specific studies, and specimens should be taken only from patients who are properly identified. Those ordering tests should be aware of the volume of blood needed and should cluster studies to avoid unnecessary heel sticks in infants. Minimal sample sizes consistent with good technique should be a laboratory goal.

Blood Bank

A full-service, accredited blood bank should be readily accessible and capable of providing a complete range of blood components as well as fresh blood for exchange transfusions. If neonates are being treated, the capability of providing small volumes of blood, with careful attention to "dead space" in the system (tubing, filter volume) and minimal waste, is necessary. Provision for an autologous transfusion program is highly desirable, especially for support of a scoliosis surgery program. Leukocyte transfusion capability is recommended to support an intensive care newborn service or a hematology or oncology service. Minor crossmatch and/or lectin screening for T-activation is strongly encouraged. Detection and identification of red blood cell antibodies are similar in principle to methods for adults; but nuances and frequency variations should be appreciated, and a knowledgeable consultant should be accessible.

Chemistry

In many tertiary units, laboratories for performing chemical tests are located in the newborn ICU area to enhance efficiency. Chemical tests should be based on micro methods, and there should be a knowledge of interfering substances. A small sample cannot be made large simply by dilution, without attention to technical considerations of the specific test. Blood gas and pH studies on arterial or arterialized capillary specimens should be maintained anaerobically, kept cool, and tested within 30 minutes of sample procurement. Results should be adjusted for the patient's hemoglobin level and temperature.

Reliable sweat testing methods should be done by pilocarpine iontophoresis. At least 50 mg of sweat must be obtained for satisfactory analysis of sodium and chloride levels. It is doubtful that a laboratory performing fewer than 12 sweat tests a year can have confidence in the results of these tests.

Tests for therapeutic drug monitoring and toxic chemical ingestion should be provided or be accessible at all times, at least in the region served. Testing for concentrations of therapeutic drugs, including antimicrobial agents, should be integrated with dose and administration time data, including "peak and trough" times for individual agents. Tests should be available for the agents commonly used in pediatrics, such as antimicrobial agents, theophylline, and phenytoin.

Cytogenetics

Modern technology, including that for cell synchronization/ high resolution karyotyping and identification of the fragile X chromosome (requiring folate-deficient media) as a marker of a unique mental retardation syndrome, should be available. The laboratory should have facility with both blood and tissue specimens; the availability of rapid chromosomal studies on bone marrow is highly desirable for assisting with major management decisions in neonatology units. Chromosomal analysis of neoplastic cells, particularly leukemic cells, is becoming increasingly important for predictive purposes and for monitoring the course of subjects under therapy; this analysis requires sophisticated techniques.

The results of chromosomal studies should be interpreted by an expert and reported in combination with relevant clinical data.

Hematology

Reporting and interpretation of hematologic data should reflect a knowledge of normal and abnormal hematopoiesis in infants and children. There should be access to expert pediatric hematopathology consultation for patients suspected of having leukemia, and material from these patients should be saved for confirmatory and additional studies, if indicated.

Micro sample techniques and modern molecular marker studies are necessary for thorough evaluation and monitoring of congenital and acquired abnormalities of coagulation.

Microbiology

Rapid identification of organisms and/or definition of antibiotic sensitivities of pathogens is essential for study of cerebrospinal fluid and blood from children with suspected bacterial sepsis. Special awareness, experience, and techniques are required for identification and antibiotic sensitivity testing of organisms such as *Haemophilus influenzae, Streptococcus pneumoniae, Neisseria meningitidis*, and group B streptococcus, which are commonly isolated from sick children. Methods for removal of antibiotics from specimens of body fluids are essential for evaluation of the treated patient.

Nonculture techniques, such as counterimmunoelectrophoresis, enzyme-linked immunosorbent assays, and fluorescent antibody methods, facilitate rapid detection and specific identification of infectious agents, including viruses.

Anatomic Pathology

Anatomic pathology is best provided by a pathologist trained and interested in pediatric pathology. Interpretation of anatomic findings must be based on knowledge of normal growth and development of infants and children, and consideration should be given to genetic implications associated with certain diagnoses. A well-defined approach to examination of tumors, important biopsy material, and specimens from an autopsy is essential so that important information is not missed by those who do not routinely perform these studies. All diagnoses of malignant neoplasia and diagnoses of other serious disorders such as Hirschsprung's disease, biliary atresia, and storage diseases should be confirmed by an experienced pediatric pathologist.

Tertiary pediatric care must be monitored through a system, including an autopsy service skilled in pediatric pathology and characterized by a genuine interest in pathogenesis of pediatric disorders and the complications of therapy and monitoring.

To enhance accuracy and efficiency, certain specimens may be sent to an outside laboratory if the test results are not urgently needed.

Table 6

Representative Rapid Response Testing and Response Times*

Test	Response Time*† (in minutes)
BUN	30
Blood ammonia	30
Blood gas and pH	15
CBC	15
Calcium	30
Coagulation studies	45
Dilantin	30
Electrolytes Cl, Na, K, HCO_3	30
Glucose	30
Iron	30
SGOT	30
Salicylate	30
Serum amylase	30
Serum bilirubin	30
Spinal fluid study (complete)	30
Theophylline	60
Type and crossmatch	60

*This table is not intended for use as a source of response time standards.

†Time lapse between laboratory's receipt of specimen and availability of results through computer.

Chapter 17

SPECIALIZED SUPPORT SERVICES

Respiratory Therapy

Respiratory therapy has emerged as a powerful weapon for the care of children with various respiratory diseases. The spectrum of respiratory care within the hospital includes administration of various aerosol agents, maneuvers to facilitate clearance of excessive secretions from the airways to prevent or treat atelectasis and pneumonia (e.g., chest clapping and percussion, segmental bronchial drainage, sterile airway suctioning, and incentive spirometry), oxygen enrichment and humidification of inspired air, and ventilator management. Diagnostically, respiratory therapists may perform arterial puncture for blood samples they then analyze for pH, PCO_2, and PO_2; perform bedside and laboratory-based pulmonary function tests from the simplest to the most sophisticated; and play a role in the attachment and operation of various monitoring devices (e.g., impedance pneumography, heart rate monitors, central venous pressure recording, transcutaneous PO_2 and PCO_2 monitoring, and ear oximetry).

Although none of these skills is unique to pediatrics, the challenge is far greater in pediatrics than in adult patients. Equipment size and type must extend from that applicable for the premature infant to that for the adolescent. In the small child, gentleness and persistence are required to overcome fear.

The therapist must be prepared to teach the child and his or her family certain techniques that may be required after discharge from the hospital and be prepared to monitor the efficacy of therapy on an outpatient basis.

Considerable skill is required in working with other professionals, including nurses, physical therapists, occupational therapists, and others, so efficient and well integrated care is given in the correct order, at the right time, and with as little patient exhaustion as possible.

Personnel

A department of respiratory therapy must be directly supervised by a registered respiratory therapist and have as medical director a physician with knowledge of intensive care, respiratory physiology, and respiratory therapy. Generally, a pulmonologist or anesthesiologist may have the requisite background and skills. In a children's hospital, the pediatric focus is routine. However, problems arise in general hospitals in which newborn infants and children comprise a minority of the patients. The interests of these young patients can be safeguarded only by pediatricians on the staff who will insist on the necessary pediatric expertise and equipment. Possible solutions include a pediatrician with the requisite pulmonary background functioning as associate medical director and a cadre of child-oriented respiratory therapists. Lines of responsibility between nursing staff and respiratory therapists also must be clear.

Equipment

Modern hospital requirements include oxygen, compressed air, and vacuum outlets in every unit in which acutely or severely ill patients are to be housed. Aerosol medications should be delivered by compressed air unless there is a specific need for oxygen. Appropriate numbers of portable oxygen cylinders must be available for oxygen-dependent patients in transit to and from the operating room, intensive care unit, emergency room, radiology department, or various laboratories.

The respiratory therapy department must be responsible for the maintenance and repair of its equipment. Nosocomial infections are an expanding threat as increasingly invasive and heroic therapy is attempted in debilitated or immunosuppressed patients. Strict rules and schedules must be established for regular sterilization of reusable equipment and for replacement of tubing and other discardable items. Regular sampling of potentially infected equipment by culturing water supplies and other critical areas of respiratory therapy,

testing, and monitoring equipment should be carried out by
an infection control team within the hospital.

Nutrition Services

An adequate intake of calories, protein, and specific nutrients plays a key role in the maintenance of body integrity,
growth, and restoration to health in childhood and adolescence. Nutrition adequacy is necessary as an adjunct to
therapy to support nonspecific defenses against infection and
the integrity of the immune system. Adequate food intake
is needed to counter the adverse affects of some therapeutic
regimens. Selective diets are essential to the management of
certain metabolic disorders, such as diabetes mellitus or
phenylketonuria. Food also plays an important role in the
emotional support of a child.

The hospital undertaking the care of children and adolescents should provide a range of dietary and nutrition services
for optimal treatment. These can be incorporated into the
medical and nursing care program by the dietary staff and
nutrition support team.

Nutrition Evaluation Services

Diet

Initial screening for patients at increased risk of a nutrition
problem may be facilitated with questionnaires concerning
food habits and a review of key anthropometric data (height,
weight) and laboratory data (hemoglobin, mean corpuscular
volume, and so forth). Evaluation of the diet includes not
only food intake during hospitalization but evaluation of the
usual diet prior to hospitalization to identify any preexisting
problems. It also is important to ensure an appropriate diet
after discharge, whether it is therapeutic or a continuation
of the regular diet.

The 24-hour recall of food intake or a usual day's intake

can be obtained from the mother or primary caretaker, or from the child directly if he or she is able to provide accurate information. A useful technique is to obtain a 7-day frequency of "protective foods" (protein sources, fresh fruit, vegetables, and foods containing vitamin A and iron). More specific data can be obtained through the use of a written record of 3- or 7-day food intake. A dietitian will convert the intake information to nutrients using food composition tables and evaluate the diet in terms of meeting the nutrient requirements for age. Special food consumption tables are available for the dietary management of a variety of inborn errors and other metabolic disorders.

A comprehensive dietetic library of these reference materials is required, as well as the services of a registered dietitian. Diet evaluation can suggest an approach to the improvement of nutrition status by use of accustomed and preferred foods.

Nutrition Status

Assessment of nutrition status should be an integral part of any initial medical or surgical work-up and long-term follow-up. This can be performed by the physician, nurse, or dietitian who has had inservice training and should provide data useful in planning for nutrition management or restoration, as well as a baseline for future comparison.

The hospital must supply the equipment and reference material for the following measurements:

1. Weight: lever beam balances plus calibrating weights.
2. Length: length board with fixed head board and sliding foot board.
3. Height: fixed height stick with sliding headpiece, preferably attached to vertical wall.
4. Arm circumference: flexible metal, fiberglas, or plastic tape.
5. Fatfold: Lange caliper or Harpenden caliper.
6. Growth charts and reference data for height, length, and weight from the National Center for Health Statistics.
7. Fatfold and arm circumference reference data.[1,2]

Anthropometry is inexpensive, can be performed by nonmedical staff, and detects mild to moderate, and severe protein-energy malnutrition.

Clinical Examination

The observation of nutritional deficiency is an integral part of the physical examination by the physician. Some hospital dietitians are trained to recognize those signs which correlate closely with nutritional deficiency.

Biomedical Assessment

Biochemical documentation of nutritional deficiency should not be carried out indiscriminately. It should be done selectively to confirm clinical evidence of deficiency or to evaluate further a patient with consistently poor intake. Patients with protein-energy malnutrition frequently have associated, specific deficiencies. In addition, patients taking therapeutic agents which are known to induce deficiencies (e.g., isoniazid, folic acid antagonists) also should be evaluated for specific nutrient deficiencies.

Nutrition and Dietary Services

Problems

The hospitalized child may be emotionally upset because of separation from the family, particularly from the mother. New surroundings, unfamiliar routines and foods, and fears about the illness and procedures contribute to the child's anxieties. Age, severity of illness, and the child's ability to cope with the new situation influence adjustment to the hospital. The young or developmentally delayed child may be unable to manipulate the utensils and/or the food because of weakness, physical restraints, or confinement to bed. Regressive behavior may cause a child who was self-feeding to demand to be fed or to be given a bottle.

Approaches

The success of nutrition care depends on the acceptance of food by the young patient. Treatments (e.g., chest physiotherapy, painful procedures) which interfere with appetite, eating, or retention of food should not be scheduled close to mealtimes. Parents should be encouraged to visit at mealtimes, especially for infants and toddlers. Whenever possible, the assistance of volunteer or surrogate parents during mealtime may increase food intake. For children who are ambulatory, family-style group eating in pleasant surroundings (e.g., in the playroom) free from medical treatment and rounds could encourage better food intake. Provision of culturally appropriate foods can be an important factor in increasing intake. Toddlers should be offered finger foods attractively served. Especially for adolescent patients, self-selection of menus and provision of facilities for preparation of snacks encourage food intake.

Parent and Patient Education

The hospital can and should provide nutrition education for the patient and the family. There should be a space for conferences and for food preparation demonstrations where both patient and parents can learn. This would be particularly useful for instruction in therapeutic or modified diets, e.g., for children with diabetes or inborn errors of metabolism. The goal is to assist parents and children to comply with instructions for appropriate nutrition care at home. Follow-up instructions should be provided in written form.

Nutrition Support Services

Secondary and tertiary care hospitals which admit pediatric patients with serious illnesses, particularly in the categories of gastroenterology, oncology, anorexia nervosa, and gastrointestinal surgery, frequently require the services of a nutrition support team. These teams are multidisciplinary in composition, can evaluate nutrition status and deficits, and have the capability of nutrition support and rehabilitation by oral, intravenous, or total parenteral nutrition essential in combatting "hospital malnutrition." Trained personnel, including a nutritionist and/or dietitian, nurse, pharmacist, and physician are needed, as is a reliable biochemistry laboratory.

A comprehensive pediatric hospital service must provide nutrition and dietary services that include the capabilities for nutrition assessment, diet evaluation, biochemical analyses for nutrients, and treatment modalities which include oral as well as total parenteral nutrition. Nutrition and dietary services also should be an integral part of ambulatory programs. The challenge is not only to treat current nutrition problems but also to prevent future problems. Improved food intake and nutrition status are most effective and inexpensive adjuncts to therapy and restoration to health.

Pharmacy

The hospital pharmacy should be under the direction of a registered pharmacist and should meet the standards of the Joint Commission on Accreditation of Hospitals.

The medical staff is required to have a pharmacy and therapeutics committee. This committee should have at least one pediatrician as a member to ensure that the special pharmacologic requirements of infants and children are met. The hospital staff also should be represented on this committee, which has a special educational role in the hospital. The hospital formulary should be reviewed annually by this committee, and the pediatric department should be consulted on proposed revisions.

The pharmacy should be staffed with adequate personnel to ensure that drugs are dispensed efficiently on a routine basis and are available immediately for use in emergencies. Commonly used drugs and emergency medications may be dispensed directly from nursing stations, but there must be access to the main pharmacy 24 hours a day. Pharmacy services which are advantageous for pediatric patients should be available; these include packaging in unit or individual doses and the ability to formulate and stock alternative dose forms or concentrations useful for pediatric patients.

A vertical flow, laminar air flow hood, or sterile room is essential to any hospital in which intravenous additives, total parenteral nutrition, or cancer chemotherapy drugs are used.

Research, experimental, and nonformulary drugs should be dispensed by and under the control of the pharmacy.

The pharmacy also may function as a drug and poison information center.

The pharmacy staff should be actively involved in professional education concerning clinical pharmacology. This education should be directed to nurses, pharmacists, physicians, and other health care providers; and it should involve drug reactions, drug interactions, toxicology, therapeutic drug monitoring, critical review of therapeutic literature, proper drug administration, new drugs, and new formulations of old drugs.

In the future, the hospital pharmacy will need access to up-to-date computer facilities, including information resources and drug utilization data. The pharmacy computer system should be integrated with other hospital data bases, especially laboratory and drug administration information. This system should be capable of monitoring patient drug profiles and drug interactions and reactions. This information should be part of patient-oriented therapeutic consultation activities conducted by trained clinical pharmacists. If possible, the clinical pharmacy should be under the direction of a trained physician clinical pharmacologist. Whether or not a physician clinical pharmacologist is available, clinical pharmacy activities should be coordinated with the medical and nursing staffs to improve the safety, efficacy, and cost effectiveness of drug therapy. This interaction requires reorientation of traditional pharmacy roles toward more direct patient care, continuing education of hospital pharmacy staff, or recruitment of pharmacists with formal clinical training or advanced pharmacy degrees (master's or doctorate).

The modern automated pharmacy can generate data regarding the potentially excessive or prolonged use of expensive antibiotics and other agents, and thus contribute to efforts to reduce the cost of care.

Rehabilitative Medicine

Rehabilitation services, which traditionally include occupational therapy and physical therapy, should be under the direct supervision of a physiatrist. Speech therapy may be an integral part of the rehabilitation service or may be an independent division.

The size of a hospital inpatient/outpatient program and the character of the patient population served will dictate the need for a full-service rehabilitation medicine department, which usually would include divisions of physical therapy, speech therapy, and occupational therapy. There are subspecialty areas related to infants' and children's therapy within these divisions. In large pediatric services, especially those with a major surgical component and/or chronically ill patients, there is a need for professionals with specialized rehabilitation training. If the limited size of a hospital makes it impractical to have a rehabilitation medicine department, consultants should be available.

Inservice education programs for students, residents, and health professionals of all disciplines represented on a rehabilitation health team should be the director's responsibility.

Physical Therapy

Physical therapists are required by law to have a written order by a licensed physician before they may attend a hospitalized patient. They may be helpful both in treatment and evauation of the severity of a problem; therefore, they should consult on and participate in the management of selected cases with joint and soft tissue injury or disease. The physical therapy department should have the necessary equipment to be able to make orthotics for correct positioning of joints.

Occupational Therapy

Occupational therapists are registered and, in most states, are licensed. When licensed, they are not required to have a physician's prescription for diagnosis or treatment. They are a valuable asset in diagnosing and treating mentally and physically handicapped children who have sensory motor-integration problems. An acute care hospital has little need for these services. However, they are essential in an outpatient program, especially one dealing with handicapped children, and in a chronic care hospital.

Speech Therapy

Speech therapists are not required to have physician supervision and may diagnose and treat independently. As with occupational therapy, the need for speech therapy depends on the type of patient service. Most speech therapy is done on an outpatient basis. Speech therapists with special training in infant development are particularly helpful because they can help evaluate sucking, swallowing, and feeding disorders and, when appropriate, recommend intervention strategies to minimize these difficulties. Parents and nurses can be taught these techniques.

References

1. Committee on Nutrition: Pediatric Nutrition Handbook, ed. 2. Elk Grove Village, Illinois: American Academy of Pediatrics, 1985.
2. Tanner, J.M., and Whitehouse, R.H.: Standards for subcutaneous fat in British children. Brit. Med. J., 1:446, 1962.

Bibliography

Foman, S.J.: Infant Nutrition, ed. 2. Philadelphia: W.B. Saunders, 1974.

Committee on Dietary Allowances, Food and Nutrition Board: Recommended Dietary Allowances, ed. 9, revised. Washington, D.C.: National Academy of Sciences, 1980.

U.S. Department of Agriculture. Composition of Foods, Agriculture Handbook No. 8. Washington, D.C.: Government Printing Office, 1963.

Suskind, R.M., and Varma, R.N.: Assessment of nutritional status of children. Pediatrics in Review, 5:195, 1984.

Moskawitz, S.T., Pereira, G., Spitzer, A., et al.: Prealbumin as a biochemical marker of nutritional adequacy in premature infants. J. Pediat., 102:749, 1983.

Pitkin, R.M.: Assessment of nutritional status of mother, fetus and newborn. Amer. J. Clin. Nutr., 34:658, 1981.

Chapter 18

AIR AND GROUND TRANSPORTATION

Optimal Characteristics of Pediatric Air and Ground Transport System

An optimal pediatric transport system combines both air and ground ambulances into a flexible, coordinated system. Three factors combine to justify such a system.

1. A pediatric transport system must transport a critical number of patients to maintain the skills of the team members and to be cost effective. The speed of air transport is necessary for the optimal care of many critically ill children, but the responsibility to serve all hospitals also necessitates the use of ground ambulances.

2. Changing weather and traffic conditions frequently restrict the mode of transport to either air or ground ambulance.

3. A pediatric transport system should be capable of responding to any call with a mode that is the least costly but still consistent with high quality medical care.

Aside from the mode of transportation, other important aspects of an effective pediatric transport system include

1. Effective communication between receiving and referring hospitals and the transport vehicles.

2. Feedback and outreach programs to promote the coordination of care between the receiving hospital, the referring hospital, and the transport system.

3. Data collection to evaluate and support feedback and outreach programs.

4. Stringently controlled protocols dealing with (a) selection of vehicles or aircraft appropriate for a given pediatric transport, (b) specific clinical situations, and (c) specific nonclinical situations such as vehicle failure and requests of family members to ride in the transport vehicle.

5. A cost accounting and billing office to provide a billing system, establish fees, and provide relationships with state agencies and third party payers.

6. Medical direction and control to coordinate patient care during transport, follow-up responsibilities, outreach responsibilities, and data collection.

7. A management and communications center staffed day and night by trained dispatchers, which facilitates communication among the receiving hospital, the referring hospital, the transport team, and ancillary support services such as security personnel.

8. Vehicles that meet established specifications for size, design, climate control, safety, and power sources.

9. A transport team available at all times and trained in intensive care and aeromedical and ground transport.

10. Self-contained, mobile intensive care equipment.

Indications for Transport

In general, a patient should be transferred when, in the physician's judgment, the referring hospital lacks the facilities and/or the personnel to provide optimal care. Referrals are made and accepted based on the judgment of the referring physician rather than on a specific set of criteria. Physician judgment has proven to be a more effective basis for transport than specific medical indications because it often may be difficult to ascertain the true condition of the patient over the telephone, and indications for transport vary considerably depending on the ability of the referring hospital to deal with a specific condition.

Criteria for Choosing the Mode of Transportation

The choice between air and ground transportation is determined by the following:

1. The optimal interhospital transport time as dictated by the nature and severity of the patient's clinical condition.
2. The stability of the patient prior to transport.
3. The region's geography.
4. Weather conditions.
5. Traffic conditions.
6. Cost.
7. Carrier availability.

The first two factors are of paramount importance. If a patient's medical condition is unstable, even a minimal shortening of transport time to the referring hospital by one mode of transportation over another may be lifesaving.

In general, for patients requiring a lifesaving procedure that can only be performed at the receiving hospital (e.g., evacuation of a patient with an intracranial hematoma), a difference in round-trip time (air *v* ground) of greater than 30 minutes may be undesirable. The choice of minimal shortening of transport time using one tolerable mode of transport versus another may be arbitrary. Cost considerations may indicate one direction and clinical considerations another. Research in this area is scanty; therefore, each system must create its own criteria for choice between modes of transportation. No firm guidelines are set at this time.

Other considerations, rather than distance *per se*, dictate the mode of transportation. These considerations indicate that an urban-suburban area without major traffic problems should have helicopter transport available, but not necessarily always utilized, for transports of greater than 20 to 30 miles, and that fixed-wing transport should be available for transports of more than 150 miles.

Data on comparable safety of the various modes of transportation are not available. All three types of vehicles appear safe if there is strict adherence to safety regulations. Surface ambulances should travel at speeds within the legal limits; the siren should be used if necessary to aid in passage through busy intersections without traffic delays. Air transport teams must observe weather restrictions. Undue haste generally is unsafe and may be counterproductive.

Personnel

The key to a successful voluntary transport system is the selection and training of the personnel involved. All personnel should be chosen for their medical skills as well as for their ability to deal sensitively with personnel at the referring hospital, with parents, and with each other.

The specific personnel used by a transport system and their duties will vary depending on the type of transport (newborn infants, older infants, or children), the relative availability of different types of medical personnel in a given system (e.g., residents, emergency medical technicians, and nurses), and the personal preferences of those organizing the program.

Although the composition of the transport team may vary from situation to situation, the presence of a medical director with overall responsibility is essential. Specific criteria should be established for determining the composition of the team to perform a given transport. Basically, the team consists of a transport physician (at least at the third-year resident level), a nurse, and a pilot or driver. Other members may include a respiratory therapist, an emergency medical technician, and a dispatcher or organizer. For patients with complex problems, either attending level pediatricians or physicians with subspecialty training in anesthesia, intensive care, or surgery should be available on a 24-hour basis to accompany the resident or nurse on transport.

Transport team members should be dually trained and competent, not only in intensive medical procedures such as monitoring but also in managing the supplies and equipment required by the transport vehicle, the physiologic effects of transport on the patient, maintenance and decontamination of equipment, and the limitations imposed by the transport environment.

Factors which affect the selection of medical transport team members are

1. Clinical competency in pediatric intensive care and experience in both surface and air transport of critically ill

children. Competence may be obtained through participation in pediatric ground or air transport, by attending a comprehensive course in pediatric transport, or both.

2. Physical and emotional limitations that may be hazardous to the team member and his or her ability to function as a team member. Limitations include mental stability; use of medications, alcohol, or tobacco; ability to withstand fatigue; susceptibility to motion sickness; physical agility; and enthusiasm and commitment.

3. Completion of a planned formal training program approved by the medical director of the system and supplemented by inservice practical training. The course should be of sufficient duration and content to cover all responsibilities related to the participation of each team member.

Pediatric Medical Transport Equipment

Selection of equipment is determined by the specific types of transports expected. The transport team should bring all equipment and drugs necessary for stabilization and transport; the referring hospital may have limited resources and capabilities. Equipment should meet the following guidelines for both air and ground transport:

1. Provide capability for life support in any type of situation.

2. Be self-contained, lightweight, and portable.

3. Be easily cleaned and maintained.

4. Be packaged to allow continuous intensive care during ingress and egress.

5. Have portable, self-contained power for twice the expected transport duration.

6. Have A-C power capability.

7. Not interfere electromagnetically with navigation and communication systems.

8. Be durable to withstand severe mechanical, thermal, and electrical stress.

Communications

Communication between the medical director and the referring physician is essential. Careful questioning usually will reveal important clues regarding the pediatric patient's true condition. This information dictates strategy regarding transfer.

All air transports must be linked directly to an air-to-ground communications system. The physician responsible for the transport should be able to communicate with the transport team at all times. Therefore, the aircraft should have a sky phone which is tied into the commercial telephone network. If the air transport connects with a ground transportation system, the ground ambulance should have direct voice communication with the local communication center and the ability to link directly with the receiving hospital. This may be accomplished by using either the Med-Com (paramedic) channels or a local or regional ambulance frequency.

The organization and mechanics of the communication system will vary with the resources available. The following components should be incorporated:

1. Receipt of request: All requests for transport should be handled promptly and personally by a pediatrician of at least third-year resident level.

2. Internal communication: A critical element is locating and informing transport personnel when a request has been received. Required personnel may not always be on the scene. The speed with which they can be located and assembled is of vital importance.

3. External communication: Where such resources are available, the transport system should be linked to a central dispatch system within the community which can provide timely voice linkages, directions, and police, fire, and emergency medical service back-up. All systems should have the capability of establishing and maintaining direct-voice communications between central dispatch, the critical care vehicle, the referring hospital, the receiving hospital, and other community disaster or emergency services. Central dis-

patch also may be responsible for automatically recording communications and for coordinating the logistics of the transport, particularly when different modes of transport (e.g., air and ground) are involved.

4. Follow-up: Follow-up should be provided to all referring physicians and hospitals on the condition of the patient at appropriate intervals. This facilitates the transfer of patients back to the referring hospital, enhances the willingness of physicians to make referrals, and provides an excellent opportunity for informal discussion and education.

Family members who are unable to accompany or follow the patient should be contacted and given a report on the child's condition as soon as possible after the transfer to relieve their anxiety. However, additional follow-up contacts are most appropriately handled by the receiving physician rather than by the transport system.

Bibliography

U.S. Department of Transportation National Highway Traffic Safety Administration and the American Medical Association Commission on Emergency Medical Services. Air Ambulance Guidelines. Washington, D.C.: U.S. Government Printing Office, 26-798/1444, 1981.

Division of Medical Sciences, National Academy of Sciences: National Research Council: Medical Requirements for Ambulance Design and Equipment, Washington, D.C.: National Research Council, 1968.

Sredl, D.M.: Airbourne Patient Care Management. St. Louis: Medical Research Associates Publications, 1983.

Dobrin, R.S., Block, B., Gilman, J.I., and Massaro, T.A.: The development of a pediatric emergency transport system. Pediat. Clin. N. Amer., 27:633, 1980.

Black, R.E., Mayer, T., Walker, M.D., Christison, E.L., Johnson, D.G., Matlak, M.E., Storrs, B., and Clark, C.: Air transport of pediatric emergency cases. New Engl. J. Med., 307:1465, 1982.

Segal, S., ed.: Manual for the Transport of High Risk Infants: Principles, Policies, Equipment, Technique. Canadian Paediatric Society, 1972. Newborn Air Transport Conference Proceedings, February 1978. Mead-Johnson Nutritional Division Publications.

Committee on Fetus and Newborn and Committee on Obstetrics: Maternal and Fetal Medicine: Guidelines for Perinatal Care. Evanston, Illinois: American Academy of Pediatrics, and Washington, D.C.: American College of Obstetricians and Gynecologists, Chapter 8, 1983.

Smith, D., and Hackel, A.: Staffing requirements for pediatric critical care transport teams. Crit. Care Med., 9:289, 1981.

Chapter 19

CHILD LIFE PROGRAMS*

One unique activity of pediatric hospital settings is the child life program. Developed over the years in children's hospitals and in hospitals affiliated with medical schools, child life programs now are found in other children's units.

Child life specialists meet the developmental, emotional, recreational, and educational needs of children. Using play and other forms of communication, they help children cope with health care experiences more positively. When children know there is a place devoted to play in the hospital, their perceptions of themselves, the illness, and the hospital may change. Thus, playrooms must be large enough to accommodate wheelchairs, traction beds, stretchers, and accompanying apparatus so that most patients can go to them.

All pediatric units should provide a child life program. Those with more than 10 patients should have a full-time child life specialist (sometimes called play therapist, recreation therapist, activity therapist). The minimum child life staff-to-child ratio should be 1:15; this includes the basic coverage for days, weekends, and holidays.

Play

Play has many important functions. It enhances feelings of self-esteem and encourages children to be part of a group. Especially important in hospitals are the opportunities to resolve fears of separation, abandonment, bodily injury, and loss of control. Play must be based on child development concepts.

Children like to play. Whether it is an infant batting a mobile or an adolescent shooting pool, play can mean fun, choices, learning, adapting, creating, and forming relationships with others. Play allows children to concentrate, to be

*Adapted from Committee on Hospital Care: Child life programs for hospitalized children, Pediatrics, 76:467, 1985.

involved, and to move in and out of situations as their medical condition allows. Children particularly like toys and activities they can control, which have moving parts, which require repetition and thus increase understanding, or which allow creativity.

The therapeutic values of play are extremely important to hospitalized children. Play dough, sand, water, clay, and finger paints—being messy—provide an acceptable outlet for feelings and for communicating nonverbally. Stroking, molding, pounding, and manipulating materials enable children to come to grips with their feelings and, with help, to attain resolution.

Medical play using actual hospital supplies and equipment is a keystone of the child life program. Observing children as they use the materials used on them enables the staff to understand how the children have internalized this information and experience. Surgical garb, syringes, and anesthesia masks are high on the list of equipment that children select for play. Opportunities for medical play should be available repeatedly.

As part of their support system, child life programs also use activities that keep children in touch with home: cooking, listening to music, housekeeping corners, and favorite toys. The provision of currently popular toys and games can help improve the image children have of hospitals. Computers and other electronic games provide the opportunity for control, choices, and competition, which help children maintain their self-esteem.

The Program

Child life programs affect many aspects of staying in hospital units: organizing playrooms, encouraging relationships between roommates in traction beds, setting up the teen lounge, relieving a parent at bedside, changing posters in the pediatric intensive care unit, playing games with a child in isolation, or checking supplies in the kitchen for a cooking project.

Children, families, and staff are reassured when they know the daily schedule of events. They should be able to depend on the playroom being open at specified hours, which should be compatible with the routine of the unit. Special events, such as puppet shows or entertainers, enrich the program and are greeted eagerly by children and parents. Children in the hospital want special attention given to holidays.

Planning a program for children with a wide range of ages and medical restraints is a challenge. Some aspects to consider include the following:

1. The safety of the toys and equipment.
2. That the toys are appropriate to developmental levels and interests.
3. That meals be served family style in the playroom.
4. That a playground or deck be developed.
5. That animals be available for watching and nurturing.

Younger children become engrossed in the process, for example, of painting or making a mobile, but adolescents will be concerned about the end product. Teen-aged patients need reassurance that their projects are worthy and that others will approve of them. Special attention should be given to each child's pace and style. For example, reflective children require more help with transitions than impulsive children, but each will need support.

More and more hospitals are turning to closed circuit television to provide entertainment and education. Programs for and by patients reveal how creatively this medium can be used—hospital news programs, filming of special events, talk shows in conjunction with a bedside telephone, and even bingo and other games from central control allow many patients to be involved. Because television noise can be a special problem to children who are not feeling well, pillow speakers are advisable. Videocassettes covering health care issues are used most effectively when appropriate staff are available to lead discussions and answer questions.

Playrooms

Playrooms should be easy to enter and understand. Children enjoy attractive, organized spaces with toys and equipment readily available. Because of the need to accommodate beds, wheelchairs, and monitoring equipment, some facilities are now allocating 50 sq ft per child. The need for electrical outlets also is influencing the planning of playrooms. Patients want access to windows and, thus, to the outside world. There must be work spaces and comfortable seating for children and adults. Open storage for toys, games, and creative supplies must be supplemented by locked cabinets that keep at hand a variety of items. Children's art should be displayed on boards and frames designed for that purpose.

Child Life Specialists

Degrees in child development, education, or therapeutic recreation are now being supplemented in some colleges by courses and practicum experiences on working with children in health care settings. Child life specialists must have nurturing skills, an understanding of human growth and development and of children under stress, and experience in the psychosocial care of children and adolescents in hospitals. Ability to plan and organize playrooms or to improve environments, communication skills, and group work techniques are other skills necessary to the work. The use and supervision of students and volunteers allow better coverage of units and help to spread the philosophy.

Working with Other Staff

Child life specialists should receive a morning report from the nurse in charge and attend morning rounds several times a week; they always should attend patient care conferences. Significant observations by the child life staff should be shared and, when indicated, written in the patient's chart. In hospitals with resident training programs, the child life specialist can model developmental and psychosocial techniques and provide inservice education.

The child life staff should be on the committees dealing with child development and patient care issues and should work closely with the social service and psychiatry departments in the care of children and/or families experiencing particular difficulties.

School

Education is such an important part of each child's life that continuation of schooling in the hospital is an accepted aspect of pediatric services. Adolescents particularly are apt to worry about "getting behind," and indeed want to go to school and to evening "study hall." The time lapse between admission and institution of schooling should be as short as possible. This is particularly important for patients with such conditions as malignancies, cystic fibrosis, or asthma, who may come to the hospital frequently for relatively short stays. Many chronically ill children now come to the hospital with homework assignments.

Some hospitals have been able to work successfully with a local school system to provide teachers on permanent assignment or for individual patients. Others have classrooms and employ their own teachers. School assignments are accomplished, and hospital personnel can provide lessons/lectures on aspects of illness or hospital services. Teaching machines, computers, and telephone teaching have added new dimensions to the education process.

Teachers must be part of the patient care team and participate in rounds, conferences, and seminars. School participation should be recorded in the patient's chart.

Collaboration with the regular school is essential. Reports and/or telephone contact must be made on discharge; the hospital teacher frequently is the best person to speak to the regular school teacher about a patient's illness and special needs.

Bibliography

Azarnoff, P., and Flegal, S.: A Pediatric Play Program. Springfield, Illinois: Charles C Thomas, 1975.

Lindquist, I.: Therapy Through Play. London: Arlington Books Ltd., 1977.
Plan, E.: Working with Children in Hospitals. Chicago: Yearbook Medical Publishers, Inc., 1971.
Thompson R.H., and Stanford, G.: Child Life in Hospitals: Theory and Practice. Springfield, Illinois: Charles C Thomas, 1981.

Some College Programs with a Major in the Child Life Field

Wheelock College (graduate and undergraduate programs), Boston, Massachusetts
Utica College of Syracuse University, Utica, New York
Mills College, Oakland, California
Northeastern Illinois University, Chicago, Illinois
Edgewood College, Madison, Wisconsin
University of Akron, Akron, Ohio

Other Publications

The following publications are available through the Association for Care of Children in Hospitals, 3615 Wisconsin Avenue, N.W., Washington, D.C. 20016:
Directory of Child Life Activity Programs in North America
Directors of Child Life Activity Practicum Experiences in North America (1981)
The Hospitalized Child Bibliography (1979)
Child Life Activities: An Overview (1980)
Ideas for Activities with Hospitalized Children (1982)
Guidelines for the Development of Child Life Programs for the Personnel Conducting Programs of Therapeutic Play for Pediatric Patients (1980)
Hospital School Programs: Guidelines and Directory (1981)
Child Life Position Statement (revised 1983)

Chapter 20

VOLUNTEER SERVICES

Voluntarism is one of the highest attributes of a civilized society. The dedication and enthusiasm of carefully screened and well-placed hospital volunteers can extend the services of staff throughout the hospital and reflect into the community as well.

Volunteers can assist in almost every area of the hospital— feeding and rocking infants; chasing toddlers; playing games; delivering mail; escorting patients; staffing the information desk; maintaining equipment and supplies; landscaping; serving as registrars, receptionists, clerks, typists, or research aides; serving in emergency rooms, gift shops, libraries, playrooms, parking lots, laboratories, medical records, or waiting rooms—in almost any supportive capacity. They bring good cheer and a special kind of caring.

For example, one major pediatric hospital has 300 active volunteers who serve in more than 50 hospital locations on a weekly basis and represent an annual productive-hour equivalent of nearly 20 full-time employees. This reflects a service donation conservatively estimated at $236,000 for a single year. Many people who cannot serve inside the hospital enrich this pediatric program by providing handcrafted toys, infant layettes, holiday decorations and gifts, and craft and playroom supplies on a regular basis. Their donations represent thousands of dollars annually. The good will quotient of donated services and goods cannot be measured.

Channeling this kind of spirit into satisfying and useful service in a child health care setting requires the highest standards of human resource management. Sound management is as essential for volunteers as for salaried staff. However, it needs to be recognized that volunteer hours and staff hours are not comparable. Because most volunteers serve only a fraction of the work week and lack the continuity of paid staff, management logistics increase. Problems can be avoided if all prospective volunteers and all staff who need volunteers rely on an established department of volunteer services to screen, select, orient, and place all volunteers. No staff member should promise placement or accept responsibility for a volunteer except through standard procedures. This ensures equal opportunity, safe practices, and quality service.

A volunteer department with a full-time director (1) serves to protect the institution, children, and parents from inappropriate individuals and services; (2) determines which programs are feasible, practical, and productive; (3) decides which needs can be met and which cannot; (4) assures volunteers of meaningful work; (5) assigns qualified volunteers according to the overall needs of the hospital; (6) keeps accurate records; (7) administers benefits; and (8) maintains good relations with the community.

The director of volunteers should have superior skills and experience in human resource management, program development, education and training, interviewing, supervision, problem solving, public relations, and promotion. Secretarial help is essential. Additional staff skilled in interviewing and training also may be needed. The institutional budget for a professionally managed volunteer program will be more than compensated for by thousands of hours of free service annually and an ever-expanding network of community support.

Although actual procedures may be simplified, written volunteer policies should be consistent with employee policies regarding equal opportunity, local health regulations, safety standards, liability, probation, identification and security, documentation of service, commitment, disciplinary actions, and terminations. Benefits may include free or discounted parking, meals, uniforms, tuberculosis screening, and educational opportunities.

Each prospective volunteer should be carefully screened. Volunteers represent a cross section of society, men and women representing every age, racial, ethnic, economic, social, and educational group. Their motivation to volunteer may be altruism, personal experiences, retirement, career exploration, a need for human contact, a desire to be useful, or a variety of other individual reasons. Any reservations obtained during an interview about an applicant's stability, maturity, motivation, hidden agenda, inordinate personal needs, available time, or ability to accept supervision or to follow institutional policies and procedures should serve as warning signals in the final selection. Good screening, orientation, and supervision will make the need for termination rare.

Many energetic and enthusiastic youths wish to volunteer because of an interest in health care careers. These young volunteers deserve careful orientation and close supervision; they should not be exploited or subjected to undue stress. For these reasons many hospitals set 16 years as a minimum age requirement and assign younger volunteers only to non-patient care areas.

For legal reasons, even the most qualified volunteers should not engage in direct medical care or treatment of any kind. A written job description should outline clearly what each volunteer may and may not do and specify who is responsible for direct supervision. Volunteer services should supplement, but never substitute for, the services of paid staff.

The work available should be worth the volunteer's time and effort and be of genuine help to staff. Volunteers should never be placed where staff does not acknowledge a need or have time and ability to provide supervision, encouragement, and feedback. The volunteer's total available service hours also must be sufficient to justify the staff time required for training and supervision. For this reason, many hospitals ask volunteers for a commitment of at least 100 service hours per year.

To assure confidence and competence, all volunteers deserve a thorough orientation to their role, the work environment, and the institutional philosophy and policies. Volunteers who work directly with children and parents must be selected with special care and oriented to safety standards, confidentiality, child development, and the emotional needs of sick children and their families. Training should enable volunteers to monitor their interactions and reactions to patients, families, and staff in the hospital setting. Well prepared volunteers can augment play programs, but the volunteers never should be expected to substitute for a consistent, ongoing, professionally staffed child life program.

Volunteers will remain committed when they know their service is worthwhile and appreciated. Both formal and informal recognition should be ongoing and performance related. Creative hospitalwide activities during a volunteer week, for example, can promote an annual celebration of team spirit for volunteers and staff alike. A well-managed volunteer department will increase staff awareness of the value of volunteered services and prepare volunteers who help improve child health care within the institution and the community.

Chapter 21

THE DYING CHILD

If I had a chance to be anything I wanted to be, I would be an eagle. Eagles soar with no fear, no worries. Eagles have a certain freedom that I would like to have. An eagle has the freedom to soar over God's creation and in God's heavens.*

These lines, written by a chronically ill, 15-year-old patient, provide insight into the needs of the dying. The message in these lines can serve as a basis for setting goals in the care of the dying child or youth. To provide optimum management of the dying child is a challenge to professionals; the patient's individual medical needs and the emotional needs of the child and family must be met. This requires each member of the health care team to come to terms with his or her personal feelings about death, thereby making it possible to draw on sensitive understanding and knowledge in planning the total care of the child and family. In particular, understanding that children and adults usually adapt to dying with strength and insight appropriate to their age is important for all staff members involved in delivering care to the dying child. This chapter will present guidelines for meeting the physical and psychologic needs of the dying child or adolescent in the hospital setting.

The Infant

An infant reacts to the physical stress of dying with all available physiologic reflexes, instinctively striving to maintain life.[1] Therefore, the medical care should be directed to keeping the dying infant as comfortable as possible. Because the infant will respond eagerly to the warmth of touch and to the satisfaction of sucking on a nipple, these comforting experiences should be provided as often as possible. Medica-

*From Mark Willian, "To Be Free," used with permission of the parents.

tions for pain or to assure rest should be used to comfort the infant when indicated. Parents will need support as they struggle with feelings of helplessness and watch their infant decline and die; they should be encouraged to hold or touch and to personally take care of their infant as often as possible.

The Young Child

Young children, toddlers, and preschool-aged children usually will react indirectly to their impending death by responding to the reaction of their parents. The dying child will fear being separated from his or her parents or may fear that hospitalization is a punishment for wrongdoing. To minimize these reactions, parents should be encouraged to spend as much time as possible with the child. The child also should be allowed to have with him or her familiar toys, blankets, or other important possessions from home; these items can help counteract the strange hospital environment and the physical discomforts. If the preschool-aged child asks about his or her illness, these questions should be answered honestly and simply. It is unrealistic to expect young children to understand much about an illness, and they will indicate by their questions what they can handle.[2]

The School-aged Child

The grade school child is developing the abilities to understand a diagnosis and prognosis and is able to grasp the idea that he or she might die. His or her questions also must be answered with simple, basic explanations. When the child asks about the prognosis, a firm but general answer should be given. Care should be taken to assure the dying school-aged child that the illness, hospitalization, and treatments are not punishments for wrongdoing. Parents of a dying school-aged child should be encouraged to participate in the care of their child as much as possible. As does any child, the dying school-aged child easily accepts care, comfort, and understanding offered by his or her parents.

The Adolescent

The adolescent, who normally develops independence from the family and focuses instead on strong peer relations, is suddenly faced with changes in psychologic and physical needs when seriously ill. His or her peer group tends to reject the dying adolescent, thus failing him or her in attempts to cope with the illness. This is probably because of the adolescent's inability to handle the death of a friend, which evokes feelings of vulnerability and fragility regarding his or her own life. Thus, dying adolescents have to increase dependence on themselves and their families.[3] This may make them feel angry toward themselves, their families, and their friends.

Dying adolescents should be given every opportunity to take care of themselves. When care by others is needed, it should be given without fuss, thereby decreasing the adolescent's feelings of dependency and inadequacy. Dying adolescents should be considered part of the health care team and should be included in the medical management planning. They should be educated honestly regarding their condition; questions usually will indicate how much information they wish to know.

The Parents

Although the professional staff should encourage the family to act as a support system for the dying child, they should be prepared to deal with a variety of parental responses and reactions to a child's illness and impending death. Feelings of denial, anger, isolation, and guilt frequently are expressed. Parents should be encouraged to ventilate these feelings, even when they are directed against the staff.

Parents also should be encouraged to participate in the decision-making process about their dying child's treatment and to help with the child's care whenever possible. Their feelings of helplessness can be minimized while giving the child natural, loving care. Parents should be allowed open visitation; and, when appropriate, beds should be made available so that they can rest to avoid exhaustion.

The professional staff can provide important, coordinated support to the parents of a dying child. Physicians should be available to answer their questions; registered nurses, social workers, and clergy should be available to provide their specialized support and information. The staff can develop and guide support groups comprised of other families to sustain bereaved parents. These support groups have many functions, such as exchanging practical information, providing an outlet for frustration, offering a social outlet for parents and siblings (thereby reducing their sense of isolation), disseminating medical information, and directing families to counseling when needed.[4]

Siblings

Siblings must be included in the family support efforts. They must be kept informed about the dying child's condition and should be encouraged to visit as often as possible to preserve ties with the patient during the long hospitalization. A good method to maintain patient-sibling communication is to encourage regular telephone contact.

Hospital Philosophy

Each hospital, in developing its individual philosophy, should address the full spectrum of needs of the dying child and his or her family. This philosophy should offer those under its care an individualized plan which includes the medical, social, and emotional needs of each dying patient and his or her family. Each hospital should evaluate ways it can provide the best total care for the dying child, including both treatment as an inpatient and support services and care in the child's home. Some parents may prefer that the child die at home, and the provision of a program of home care for the dying child should be considered by the hospital. The pros and cons of a home program need to be carefully evaluated for each child and family.

Care of a dying child or adolescent requires team management and planning, utilizing a multidisciplinary approach. Physicians, nurses, social workers, child life specialists, clergy, and other professionals each offer specialized care on an individual level. This team, working with the family, can plan for each child in a personal and comprehensive manner. Team conferences should be utilized to discuss and evaluate treatment, medical management, feelings, and problems.

Team conferences also provide the staff an opportunity to express their personal reactions and feelings. Anger, sadness, helplessness, frustration, and a sense of failure are all common reactions of professionals when faced with the loss of a patient. The staff should understand that these are normal reactions, and they should have an opportunity to express them. The staff may tend to withdraw from the dying child and his or her family because of these feelings. Therefore, a special effort should be made by the staff to make frequent visits to the child's room to offer care and support.

Hospitals also should consider follow-up care after a child's death. Support groups, correspondence by physicians and/or staff, and individual counseling for parents and/or siblings are helpful strategies for follow-up care. This care is important in assisting with the grieving process, thereby decreasing the amount of guilt, mental difficulties, and unresolved grief found in a high percentage of families following the death of a child or adolescent.

The hospital staff can help the dying child and his or her family by being sensitive to the needs of each, by understanding the developmental stage and the level of understanding of the child, and by developing strategies to offer support and care to the patient and family. Open, honest communication, optimal medical care, and compassionate concern provide the dying child and his or her family with positive last days together.

References

1. Easson, W.M.: The Dying Child. The Management of the Child or Adolescent Who is Dying, ed. 2. Springfield, Illinois: Charles C Thomas, p. 23, 1981.

2. Easson, W.M.: The Dying Child. The Management of the Child or Adolescent Who is Dying, ed. 2. Springfield, Illinois: Charles C Thomas, p. 36, 1981.
3. Easson, W.M.: The Dying Child. The Management of the Child or Adolescent Who is Dying, ed. 2. Springfield, Illinois: Charles C Thomas, p. 56, 1981.
4. Coping with Cancer. Bethesda, Maryland: National Cancer Institute, p. 107, 1980.

Bibliography

Bluebond-Langner, M.: Private Worlds of Dying Children. Princeton: Princeton University Press, 1980.

Kleinberg, S.B.: Educating the Chronically Ill Child. Rockville, Maryland. Aspen Systems Corporation, 1982.

McCollum, A.T.: The Chronically Ill Child. A Guide for Parents and Professionals. New Haven: Yale University Press, 1981.

Sahler, O.J., ed.: The Child and Death. St. Louis: C.V. Mosby Company, 1978.

Spinetta, J.J., and Deasey-Spinetta, P.M., ed.: Living with Childhood Cancer. St. Louis: C.V. Mosby Company, 1981.

Appendix A

Isolation Precautions for Hospitalized Children

Recommendations in the *Red Book* for isolation of patients are in accordance with the most recent guidelines of the Centers for Disease Control (CDC).* These guidelines were developed by the CDC in conjunction with a consultative group of experts, which included pediatric infectious disease specialists, hospital epidemiologists, and infection control nurses. The guidelines incorporate two major changes: (1) two systems of isolation, category specific (e.g., enteric) and disease specific, have been developed; (2) for category specific, the categories of isolation have been changed and now total seven (strict, contact, respiratory, AFB, enteric, drainage/secretion, and blood/body). The new disease-specific recommendations are an alternative system which allows individualization of infection control measures for the disease in question; but, as a result, the recommendations are more complex for hospital personnel to implement.

The CDC has not recommended which system should be used in hospitals. The category-specific system is simple, indicates measures that are generally appropriate for each disease, and provides appropriate guidelines. Recommendations in the *Red Book* are primarily category specific. Exceptions include acute respiratory infections, in which the risks of spread and the consequences of infection warrant more specific recommendations. Alternatively, hospitals may elect to adopt the disease-specific system for all diseases.

Infection control practices in intensive care units (ICU) and those for newborn infants and young children frequently have to be modified to accommodate special circumstances, particularly those pertaining to isolation in a private room. Separate isolation rooms frequently are not available in ICU's, and newborn nurseries may not be desirable for the optimal care of critically ill patients. An isolation area can be defined within the ICU by curtains, partitions, or other markers, **if airborne transmission is not likely**. For newborn infants, separate iso-

---

*Garner, J.S., and Simmons, B.P.: Guidelines for isolation precautions in hospitals. Infect. Control, 1983;4(suppl.):245.

lation rooms frequently are not indicated if the following conditions are met:

1. An adequate number of nursing and medical personnel are on duty and have sufficient time for appropriate hand washing.

2. Sufficient space is available for a 4- to 6-ft aisle or area between newborn infant stations.

3. An adequate number of sinks for hand washing are available in each nursery room or area.

4. Continuing instruction is given to personnel about the mode of transmission of infections.

When a private room is mandated (e.g., an infant with chickenpox), a forced air incubator is **not** a substitute for a private room because these incubators do not filter the air discharged into the environment. Another modification that may be necessary for newborn infants and children during outbreaks is the cohorting of patients. Decisions of this type should be made in conjunction with the hospital's infection control and nursery directors. In all instances, **frequent and appropriate hand washing between patient contact is always necessary.**

The specifications for the seven categories of isolation are provided on instruction cards, which should be posted conspicuously in the immediate vicinity of the patient. The information on the cards is given below and on the following pages. Color-coded cards, which help to draw attention to the precautions in effect, can be obtained.

Strict Isolation

Visitors—Report to Nurses' Station Before Entering Room

1. Masks are indicated for all persons entering room.
2. Gowns are indicated for all persons entering room.
3. Gloves are indicated for all persons entering room.
4. **Hands must be washed after touching the patient or potentially contaminated articles and before taking care of another patient.**
5. Articles contaminated with infective material should be discarded or bagged and labeled before being sent for decontamination and reprocessing.

Diseases Requiring Strict Isolation‡

Diphtheria, pharyngeal
Lassa fever and other viral hemorrhagic fevers, such as Marburg virus disease§
Plague, pneumonic
Smallpox§
Varicella (chickenpox)
Zoster, localized in immunocompromised patient, or disseminated

Contact Isolation

Visitors—Report to Nurses' Station Before Entering Room

1. Masks are indicated for those who come close to patient.
2. Gowns are indicated if soiling is likely.
3. Gloves are indicated for touching infective material.
4. **Hands must be washed after touching the patient or potentially contaminated articles and before taking care of another patient.**
5. Articles contaminated with infective material should be discarded or bagged and labeled before being sent for decontamination and reprocessing.

Diseases or Conditions Requiring Contact Isolation‖

Acute respiratory infections in infants and young children, including croup, colds, bronchitis, and bronchiolitis caused by respiratory syncytial virus, adenovirus, coronavirus, influenza viruses, parainfluenza viruses, and rhinovirus
Conjunctivitis, gonococcal, in newborn infants
Diphtheria, cutaneous
Endometritis, group A streptococcus
Furunculosis, staphylococcal, in newborn infants
Herpes simplex, disseminated, severe primary or neonatal

‡A private room is indicated for strict isolation; in general, however, patients infected with the same organism may share a room. See Guideline for Isolation Precautions in Hospitals* for details and for how long to apply precautions.

§A private room with special ventilation is indicated.

‖A private room is indicated for contact isolation; in general, however, patients infected with the same organisms may share a room. During outbreaks, infants and young children with the same respiratory clinical syndrome may share a room. See Guidelines for Isolation Precautions in Hospitals* for details and for how long to apply precautions.

Impetigo

Influenza, in infants and young children

Multiply resistant bacteria, infection or colonization (any site)
with any of the following:
- Gram-negative bacilli resistant to all aminoglycosides
  that are tested. (In general, such organisms should be
  resistant to gentamicin, tobramycin, and amikacin for
  these special precautions to be indicated.)
- *Staphylococcus aureus* resistant to methicillin (or nafcil-
  lin or oxacillin if they are used instead of methicillin
  for testing)
- Pneumococcus resistant to penicillin
- *Haemophilus influenzae* resistant to ampicillin (beta-
  lactamase positive) **and** chloramphenicol
- Other resistant bacteria may be included in this isolation
  category if they are judged by the infection control team
  to be of special clinical and epidemiologic significance.

Pediculosis

Pharyngitis, infectious, in infants and young children

Pneumonia, viral, in infants and young children

Pneumonia, *Staphylococcus aureus* or group A streptococcus

Rabies

Rubella, congenital and other

Scabies

Scalded skin syndrome (Ritter's disease)

Skin, wound, or burn infection, major (draining and not covered by a dressing, or dressing does not adequately contain
the purulent material), including those infected with
Staphylococcus aureus or group A streptococcus

Vaccinia (generalized and progressive eczema vaccinatum)

Respiratory Isolation

Visitors—Report to Nurses' Station Before Entering Room

1. Masks are indicated for those who come close to patient.
2. Gowns are not indicated.
3. Gloves are not indicated.
4. **Hands must be washed after touching the patient or
   potentially contaminated articles and before taking
   care of another patient.**
5. Articles contaminated with infective material should be
   discarded or bagged and labeled before being sent for decontamination and reprocessing.

Diseases Requiring Respiratory Isolation[1]

Epiglottitis, *Haemophilus influenzae*
Erythema infectiosum
Measles
Meningitis
* bacterial, etiology unknown
* *Haemophilus influenzae*, known or suspected
* meningococcal, known or suspected

Meningococcal pneumonia
Meningococcemia
Mumps
Pertussis (whooping cough)
Pneumonia, *Haemophilus influenzae*, in children (any age)

Acid-fast Bacilli (AFB) Isolation

Visitors—Report to Nurses' Station Before Entering Room

1. Masks are indicated only when patient is coughing and does not reliably cover mouth.
2. Gowns are indicated only if needed to prevent gross contamination of clothing.
3. Gloves are not indicated.
4. **Hands must be washed after touching the patient or potentially contaminated articles and before taking care of another patient.**
5. Articles should be discarded, cleaned, or sent for decontamination and reprocessing.

Diseases Requiring AFB Isolation**

This isolation category is for patients with current pulmonary tuberculosis who have a positive sputum smear or a chest roentgenographic appearance that strongly suggests current (active) tuberculosis. Laryngeal tuberculosis also is included in this category. In general, infants and young children with pulmonary tuberculosis do not require isolation precautions because they rarely cough and their bronchial secretions con-

---

[1]A private room is indicated for respiratory isolation; in general, however, patients infected with the same organism may share a room. See Guideline for Isolation Precaution in Hospitals* for how long to apply precautions.

**A private room with special ventilation is indicated for AFB isolation. In general, patients infected with the same organism may share a room. See Guidelines for Isolation Precautions in Hospitals* for details and for how long to apply precautions.

tain few AFB compared with adults with pulmonary tuber-culosis. To protect patients' privacy, card is labeled AFB Iso-lation instead of Tuberculosis Isolation.

Enteric Precautions

Visitors—Report to Nurses' Station Before Entering Room

1. Masks are not indicated.
2. Gowns are indicated if soiling is likely.
3. Gloves are indicated for touching infective material.
4. **Hands must be washed after touching the patient or potentially contaminated articles and before taking care of another patient.**
5. Articles contaminated with infective material should be discarded or bagged and labeled before being sent for decon-tamination and reprocessing.

Diseases Requiring Enteric Precautions[††]

Amebic dysentery
Cholera
Coxsackievirus disease
Diarrhea, acute illness with suspected infectious etiology
Echovirus disease
Encephalitis (unless known not to be caused by enteroviruses)
Enterocolitis caused by *Clostridium difficile* or *Staphylococcus aureus*
Enteroviral infection
Gastroenteritis caused by
- *Campylobacter* species
- *Cryptosporidium* species
- *Dientamoeba fragilis*
- *Escherichia coli* (enterotoxic, enteropathogenic, or enteroinvasive)
- *Giardia lamblia*
- *Salmonella* species
- *Shigella* species
- *Vibrio parahaemolyticus*
- Viruses—including Norwalk agent and rotavirus

[††]A private room is indicated for enteric precautions if patient hygiene is poor. A patient with poor hygiene does not wash hands after touching infective material, contaminates the environment with infective material, or shares contaminated articles with other patients. In general, patients infected with the same organism may share a room. See Guidelines for Isolation Precautions in Hospitals* for details and for how long to apply precautions.

- *Yersinia enterocolitica*
- Unknown etiology but presumed to be an infectious agent

Hand, foot, and mouth disease

Hepatitis, viral, type A

Herpangina

Meningitis, viral (unless known not to be caused by enteroviruses)

Necrotizing enterocolitis

Pleurodynia

Poliomyelitis

Typhoid fever (*Salmonella typhi*)

Viral pericarditis, myocarditis, or meningitis (unless known not to be caused by enteroviruses)

Drainage/Secretion Precautions

Visitors—Report to Nurses' Station Before Entering Room

1. Masks are not indicated.
2. Gowns are indicated if soiling is likely.
3. Gloves are indicated for touching infective material.
4. **Hands must be washed after touching the patient or potentially contaminated articles and before taking care of another patient.**
5. Articles contaminated with infective material should be discarded or bagged and labeled before being sent for decontamination and reprocessing.

Diseases Requiring Drainage/Secretion Precautions‡‡

Infectious diseases included in this category are those that result in production of infective purulent material, drainage, or secretions, unless the disease is included in another isolation category that requires more rigorous precautions. (If you have questions about a specific disease, see the listing of infectious diseases in Table A in Guideline for Isolation Precautions in Hospitals*.)

The following infections are examples of those included in this category provided they are **not** (a) caused by multiple resistant microorganisms, (b) major (draining and not covered by a dressing, or dressing does not adequately contain the drainage) skin, wound, or burn infections, including those

---

‡‡A private room usually is not indicated for drainage/secretion precautions. See Guidelines for Isolation Precautions in Hospitals* for details and for how long to apply precautions.

caused by *Staphylococcus aureus* or group A streptococcus, or (c) gonococcal eye infections in newborn infants. See Contact Isolation if the infection is one of these three.

Abscess, minor or limited
Burn infection, minor or limited
Conjunctivitis
Decubitus ulcer, infected, minor or limited
Skin infection, minor or limited
Wound infection, minor or limited

Blood/Body Fluid Precautions

1. Masks are not indicated.
2. Gowns are indicated if soiling with blood or body fluids is likely.
3. Gloves are indicated for touching blood or body fluids.
4. **Hands should be washed immediately if they are potentially contaminated with blood or body fluids and before taking care of another patient.**
5. Articles contaminated with blood or body fluids should be discarded or bagged and labeled before being sent for decontamination and reprocessing.
6. Care should be taken to avoid needle-stick injuries. Used needles should not be recapped or bent; they should be placed in a prominently labeled, puncture-resistant container designated specifically for such disposal.
7. Blood spills should be cleaned up promptly with a solution of 5.25% sodium hypochlorite diluted 1:10 with water.

Diseases Requiring Blood/Body Fluid Precautions§§

Acquired immunodeficiency syndrome (AIDS)
Arthropodborne viral fevers (for example, dengue, yellow fever, and Colorado tick fever)
Babesiosis
Creutzfeldt-Jakob disease
Hepatitis B (including HBsAg antigen carrier)
Hepatitis, non-A, non-B

---

§§A private room is indicated for blood/body fluid precautions if patient hygiene is poor. A patient with poor hygiene does not wash hands after touching infective material, contaminates the environment with infective material, or shares contaminated articles with other patients. In general, patients infected with the same organism may share a room. See Guidelines for Isolation Precautions in Hospitals* for details and for how long to apply precautions.

Leptospirosis
Malaria
Rat-bite fever
Relapsing fever
Syphilis, primary and secondary with skin and mucous membrane lesions

Disease Specific Isolation Precautions

An instruction card with the following information has been designed to give concise information about disease-specific isolation precautions. The instruction card can be prepared by checking items and filling in blanks. After the card has been prepared, it should be displayed conspicuously near the patient who is on isolation precautions (on the door, the foot or the head of the bed, and so forth). A duplicate instruction card also may be attached to the front of the patient's chart.

Visitors—Report to Nurses' Station Before Entering Room

1. Private room indicated?   _____No
                              _____Yes

2. Masks indicated?   _____No
                              _____Yes for those close to patient
                              _____Yes for all persons entering room

3. Gowns indicated?   _____No
                              _____Yes if soiling is likely
                              _____Yes for all persons entering room

4. Gloves indicated?   _____No
                              _____Yes for touching infective material
                              _____Yes for all persons entering room

5. Special precautions   _____No
   indicated for handling   _____Yes
   blood?

6. **Hands must be washed after touching the patient or potentially contaminated articles and before taking care of another patient.**

7. Articles contaminated with _____
                                        (infective materials)
   should be discarded or bagged and labeled before being sent for decontamination and reprocessing.

Instructions

1. Locate the disease (given in Table B in Guideline for Isolation Precautions in Hospitals*), for which isolation precautions are indicated.
2. Write the disease in the blank space here:_____
3. Determine if a private room is indicated. In general, patients infected with the same organism may share a room. For some diseases or conditions, a private room is indicated if patient hygiene is poor. A patient with poor hygiene does not wash hands after touching infective material (e.g. feces, purulent drainage, or secretions), contaminates the environment with infective material, or shares contaminated articles with other patients.
4. Place a check mark beside the indicated precautions on front of the card.
5. Cross through precautions that are **not** indicated.
6. Write infective material in blank space in item 7 on front of the card.

Appendix B

Relative Importance of Equipment, Services, and Programs
in the Tertiary PICU

	Important	Desirable	Optional
General			
Category I facility			
(AMA guidelines)	X		
Regional participation	X		
Prehospital care system	X		
Transfer arrangements	X		
Transport system	X		
Communications link to			
EMS system		X	
Regional education		X	
Organization			
PICU committee	X		
Department/unit status		X	
Separate budget		X	
Delineation of physician and			
nonphysician privileges	X		
Policies for			
Nosocomial infection	X		
Safety	X		
Traffic control	X		
Parent visitation	X		
Admission and discharge			
policies	X		
Patient monitoring	X		
Life support techniques	X		
Equipment maintenance	X		
Essential equipment breakdown	X		
System of record keeping	X		
Periodic review of			
Morbidity and mortality	X		
Quality of care	X		
Safety	X		
Open admission for all staff			
physicians	X		
Medical Director			
Written definition of			
responsibilities	X		
Training and/or experience			
and expertise in intensive care	X		
Development of policies	X		
Supervision of resuscitations	X		

	Important	Desirable	Optional
Coordination of medical care		X	
Determination of patient isolation			X
Maintenance of equipment			X
Preparation of annual budget		X	
Coordination of staff education		X	
Maintenance of statistics	X		
Implementation of policy	X		
Substitute available	X		
Primary attending responsibility		X	
Right to request consultation on any PICU patient		X	
Coordination of research		X	

Physician Staff
Physicians present in hospital 24 hours

	Important	Desirable	Optional
Pediatricians	X		
Anesthesiologists		X	
Surgeons	X		
Subspecialty physicians on call	X		

Nursing Staff

	Important	Desirable	Optional
Head Nurse	X		
RN patient ratio 1:1 to 1:3 as needed	X		
Nurse orientation	X		
Nursing skills			
Recognize, interpret, record physiologic parameters	X		
Administer drugs	X		
Administer fluids and electrolytes	X		
Resuscitation	X		
Perform aspects of respiratory care	X		
Administer electronic patient monitoring	X		
Recognize psychological needs	X		

Other Team Members

	Important	Desirable	Optional
Respiratory therapist (24 hr)	X		
Biomedical technicians or equipment exchange capability (24 hr)	X		
Unit clerk (24 hr)	X		
Psychiatric support		X	
Child life specialists		X	
Clergy		X	
Social workers		X	
Nutritionists		X	

	Important	Desirable	Optional
Physical therapists		X	
Occupational therapists		X	
Supporting Services			
Laboratory	X		
Blood gas facility	X		
Radiology	X		
Blood bank	X		
Pharmacy	X		
Physical Facility: External			
Distinct unit	X		
Controlled access	X		
Adjacent to			
Elevator		X	
Emergency room		X	
Operating room		X	
Recovery room		X	
Laboratory			X
Radiology			X
Other critical care units			X
Physician on-call room	X		
Medical director's office			X
Head nurse's office			X
No through traffic	X		
Key-controlled elevators	X		
Alarm capability to central hospital to summon additional personnel	X		
Waiting room		X	
Family sleep arrangements		X	
Family counseling space	X		
Staff lounge		X	
Staff locker space		X	
Janitor's closet	X		
Clean linen storage (internal or external)	X		
Nourishment station (internal or external)	X		
Patient personal effects storage (internal or external)	X		
Clean workroom (internal or external)	X		
Soiled workroom (internal or external)	X		
Intermediate care area		X	
Physical Facility: Internal			
Patient isolation capacity	X		
Patient privacy provisions	X		

	Important	Desirable	Optional
Central station, direct patient visualization	X		
Medication station with drug refrigerator and narcotics cabinet	X		
Separate charting area			X
Conference area		X	
Staff toilet	X		
Bedpan washing facility	X		
Emergency equipment storage	X		
Hand washing facilities	X		
Patient toilet		X	
Counter and cabinet space	X		
Bedside alarm	X		
Clocks, televisions, radios, windows		X	
Access to patient's head and neck	X		
11 electrical outlets per bed	X		
14-18 electrical outlets per bed		X	
2 oxygen outlets per bed	X		
1 compressed air outlet per bed	X		
2 or more compressed air outlets per bed		X	
2 vacuum outlets per bed	X		
3 or more vacuum outlets per bed		X	
Conforming to building or federal codes			
Heating, ventilating, air-conditioning	X		
Fire safety features	X		
Electronic grounding	X		
Plumbing facilities	X		
Illumination	X		
Miscellaneous technical features	X		
Computer, microprocessor		X	
Portable Equipment			
Emergency cart	X		
Spotlight	X		
Respirators	X		
Doppler ultrasound BP device	X		
Infusion pumps including microinfusion capability	X		
Infusion controllers	X		
IV fluid warmer		X	
Defibrillator and cardioverter	X		
Suction machine (if not at bedside)	X		

	Important	Desirable	Optional
Electronic thermometers	X		
Expanded scale electronic thermometer	X		
Automated blood pressure apparatus		X	
Refractometer	X		
Otoscope/ophthalmoscope	X		
Metabolic bed scale		X	
Pressure infusors	X		
Rocking chair			X
Resuscitation bag-valve-mask device	X		
Cribs	X		
Beds	X		
Incubators	X		
Oxygen tanks	X		
Heating/cooling blankets	X		
Bilirubin lights	X		
Humidifiers	X		
Compressors	X		
Air-oxygen blenders	X		
Oxygen analyzers	X		
Servo controlled heating units with or without open crib	X		
Pacemakers	X		
EEG	X		
Transcutaneous PO_2		X	
Transcutaneous PCO_2			X
Portable transport monitor	X		
End tidal PCO_2 measurement		X	
Small Equipment			
Emergency drugs	X		
Tracheal intubation equipment	X		
Artificial airways	X		
Isolation equipment	X		
Equipment for vascular access	X		
Monitoring Equipment			
Capability for continuous monitoring of			
ECG, heart rate	X		
Respiration	X		
Temperature	X		
Arterial pressure	X		
Central venous pressure	X		
Pulmonary arterial pressure	X		
Intracranial pressure	X		
Esophageal pressure			X
3 simultaneous pressure capability	X		

	Important	Desirable	Optional
4 simultaneous pressure capability		X	
5 simultaneous pressure capability			X
Arrhythmia alarm			X

Equipment Characteristics

	Important	Desirable	Optional
High/low alarms: heart rate, respiratory rate, and all pressures			
Visible	X		
Audible	X		
Hard copy capability		X	
Electrical patient isolation	X		
Routine testing and maintenance	X		

Appendix C

TECHNICAL CONSIDERATIONS RELATING TO INTENSIVE CARE UNITS*

The environmental systems and the physical facilities in each unit must conform to local building codes and standards; state health codes; the *Minimum Requirements of Construction and Equipment for Hospitals and Medical Facilities,* which summarizes the regulations of the U.S. Department of Health and Human Services; and the *Accreditation Manual for Hospitals,* which lists the standards of the JCAH. The applicable building code and the appropriate state health code are dependent on the location of the institution. No attempt has been made to include these local regulations here. Because the federal minimum regulations and the JCAH requirements determine eligibility for Medicare and Medicaid payments, and both apply throughout the United States, these standards are the basis of the guidelines.

Although many technical details of intensive care unit construction are beyond the scope of this discussion, the following items are useful for physicians planning new units or working in existing units.

Electrical Equipment

Outlets

The minimum requirements call for two duplex outlets located on each side of the head of each bed, an outlet for television (usually high on a wall), and one duplex outlet on each other side wall for a total of 11 convenience outlets in

---

*Planning requirements and construction standards are subject to constant revisions. The reader is cautioned to consult up-to-date information before starting serious planning.

a cubicle or room. Experience indicates that 18 electrical outlets per patient more nearly provide the flexibility needed in present-day intensive therapy. All outlets, lighting fixtures, nurses' call and alarm systems, and essential services such as exhaust fans, vacuum systems, and sewer pumps, should be served by an emergency power system which will intervene within 10 seconds if the normal power system fails.

Pediatric Outlets

If pediatric patients may have contact with electrical outlets, a tamper-proof receptacle is required to limit improper access to energized contacts.

X-ray Equipment Outlets

Special x-ray equipment outlets, if used, require connection of the grounding terminal to the room grounding system. Portable, capacitative charge x-ray units can be attached to the outlets in the patient room.

Grounding

Critical care patients frequently are at high risk for electrical accidents because of indwelling catheters and pacemakers. Contact of the patient or equipment with conductive surfaces of different electrical potentials may be fatal. For this reason, electric codes call for or permit special patient isolation, ground fault circuit interrupters, and/or grounding systems in PICU areas. An equipment grounding point with one or more grounding jacks for grounding equipment is required. Because of wide variations in local electric codes, qualified counsel should be obtained when electrical isolation and the grounding of patients are being considered.

Illumination

1. Background or night lighting: low intensity lighting below the patient's bed level should allow an attendant to move safely and still not interfere with the patient's sleep.

2. Reading lights should produce a minimum of 35 ft candles at the patient's reading material. The light fixture should be located so that the beam will not be eclipsed by the head of the bed when raised and it will not interfere with intravenous poles and other equipment.

3. General illumination from an overhead fixture should provide an intensity of 20 ft candles. The lenses in this fixture should be designed to cut off the light to avoid excessive brightness in the patient's face.

4. Emergency lighting from an overhead fixture should provide a level of at least 100 ft candles at the bed for use during emergencies and treatment.

Note: Both general illumination and emergency lighting can be obtained from the same fixture. The unit is an area lighting device consisting of four 40-watt fluorescent tubes in a housing approximately 2 by 4 ft. The wiring is arranged so that two tubes light for general use and four tubes light for emergencies.

Deluxe warm or deluxe cool white fluorescent tubes produce the most natural skin colors for patient observation. These tubes may have a lower output than commercial lamps; in some instances more tubes may be required to obtain the necessary level of illumination.

Spotlights which give a high level of illumination in a small area frequently are necessary for examination and treatment. Permanently mounted wall or ceiling spotlights are difficult to adjust when the angle or distance must be changed. Portable spotlights for these procedures have greater adaptability.

Heating, Ventilating, and Air-conditioning

The federal minimum requirements include certain standards that are fundamental in facility design for new construction or modernization projects:

1. The temperature, based on individual room control, must be adjustable between 72° and 78°F (22° and 25.5°C).

2. The relative humidity must be in the range of 30% to 60%.

3. The intensive care units must have a positive air pressure relationship with the adjacent area.

4. A minimum of two air changes per hour of outdoor air must be supplied to the room.

5. A minimum of six total air changes per hour must be supplied to the room.

6. Air may be recirculated if the outdoor air requirement is met and the recirculated air passes through a two-bed filter.

7. Central make-up air systems that supply intensive care units are to be equipped with two-bed filtration equipment. *Note*: Two-bed filtration systems as specified by Standard 52-76 of the American Society of Heating, Refrigeration and Air Conditioning Engineers and Standard 680-74 of the Air-Conditioning and Refrigeration Institute call for a filter bed with an efficiency of 25% proximal (upstream) of the air-conditioning equipment and a second filter with an efficiency of 90% distal (downstream) of the fan and associated air-conditioning equipment.

8. Induction units: Hospital patient rooms frequently are air-conditioned with air supplied from induction units. With this system, air from within the room is mixed with the supply air, which does not meet the requirement of a two-bed filter system to treat recirculated air. If an induction system must be used, the units will require modification.

Materials and Finishes

The flame spread and smoke generation standards of the applicable federal and local fire codes will govern the choice of materials and finishes which can be used in the construction of facilities.

Plumbing

All plumbing systems shall be designed in accordance with the requirements of the National Standard Plumbing Code, Chapter 14. Backflow preventers (vacuum breakers) are required on certain hose connections, bedpan flushers, and laboratory sinks that may be installed.

Oxygen

Two oxygen station outlets per patient are required by the minimum federal standards. Oxygen from the hospital central storage system will be piped to the area at the head of the bed according to the standards enumerated in the National Fire Protection Association, Standard 56-F, Non-flammable Medical Gas System. Connections to the outlets will be made with keyed plugs to prevent the interchangeability of gases as specified in the Standard of the Compressed Gas Association. The transmission pressure of the oxygen pipeline is 3.5 kg/cm^2 (50 to 55 lb per sq in). Therapy equipment attached to the station outlet must contain a pressure-reducing device. A shut-off valve is required between the station outlet and the oxygen main to terminate the flow for outlet servicing, or in an emergency. An alarm system is required to warn of critical reductions in oxygen pressure.

Vacuum

The federal minimum requirements call for at least two vacuum outlets per intensive care bed. It is generally accepted that a third outlet is required, especially because a siamese connection in vacuum piping is usually unsatisfactory. All outlets should be located at the patient's head so that they are available for nasogastric, abdominal, and thoracostomy drainage, which require different levels of vacuum. A negative pressure of 50.8 cm of mercury (20 in of mercury) at the outlet will satisfy most requirements; the required pressure can be adjusted by the regulator on the receiving bottle. Pipe sizing can be critical and should conform to the Compressed Gas Association Code P-2.1.

Compressed Air

One compressed air outlet should be located at the head of each patient. For this service, air should be obtained from a clean source (such as the double filtered air-conditioning supply to PICU or to surgery) and should be compressed to a line pressure of 3.5 kg/cm^2 (50 to 55 lb per sq in) with an oil-free compressor. After leaving the compressor, the air should be filtered again, then dried in a desiccant or refrigerated drier. Conventional hospital control air usually is not acceptable because of its lack of purity and the potential hazard of an oil-oxygen explosion.

Codes and Standards

The codes and standards in the following list dictate the minimum requirements for a pediatric intensive care unit.

Minimum Requirements of Construction and Equipment for Hospitals and Medical Facilities: U.S. Department of Health and Human Services

Accreditation Manual for Hospitals: Joint Commission on Accreditation of Hospitals

State and Municipal Building Codes

State and Municipal Public Health Codes

Life Safety Code 101: National Fire Protection Association

Inhalation Anesthetics 56A: National Fire Protection Association

Respiratory Therapy 56B: National Fire Protection Association

Laboratories in Health Related Institutions 56C: National Fire Protection Association

Standard for Nonflammable Medical Gas Systems 56F: National Fire Protection Association

National Electric Code 70: National Fire Protection Association

Essential Electric Systems 76A: National Fire Protection Association

Air Conditioning and Ventilating Systems 90A: National Fire Protection Association

Code for Elevators A17.1: American National Standards Institute

Making Buildings and Facilities Accessible to the Physically Handicapped A117.1: American National Standards Institute

Energy Conservation in New Building Design 90-75: American Society of Heating, Refrigeration and Air Conditioning Engineers

Methods of Testing Air Cleaning Devices, Standard 52: American Society of Heating, Refrigeration and Air Conditioning Engineers

Standard for Air Filter Equipment, Standard 680: Air- Conditioning and Refrigeration Institute

Standard for Medical-Surgical Vacuum Systems in Hospitals, Pamphlet P-2.1: Compressed Gas Association

Laboratory Measurements of Airborne Sound Transmission, E90: American Society for Testing Materials

Classification for Determination of Sound Transmission Class, E 413: American Society for Testing Materials

National Standard Plumbing Code: National Association of Plumbing-Heating-Cooling Contractors

Safe Use of Electricity in Hospitals Code 76B: National Fire Protection Association

Appendix D

RESUSCITATION CART SUPPLIES

Cart #_____ Date_____ Time_____
Signature_____ Seal #_____

Outside Cart
_____ Cardiac back board
_____ Oxygen tanks (2)
_____ Tank wrench (1)
_____ Oxygen regulator with flowmeter (1)
_____ IV pole (1)
_____ Stethoscope (1)

Documents
_____ Equipment
_____ Resuscitation records (1)
_____ Drug dosage reference book (1)

First Drawer

Pharmacy	*Syringes*
_____ Sodium bicarbonate (1 mEq/ml)	10 ml (#4)
_____ Sodium bicarbonate (1 mEq/ml)	50 ml (#4)
_____ Epinephrine 1:10,000 (0.1 mg/ml) (at least one with 18 ga, 3½-in needle)	10 ml (#4)
_____ Calcium chloride 10% (1.36 mEq Ca^{++}/ml)	10 ml (#2)
_____ Atrophine sulfate (0.1 mg/ml)	10 ml (#2)
_____ Isoproterenol 1:50,000 (0.02 mg/ml)	10 ml (#2)
_____ Lidocaine 1% (10 mg/ml)	10 ml (#2)
_____ Dextrose 50%	50 ml (#1)
_____ Bacteriostatic sodium chloride for injection	30 ml (#2)
_____ Bacteriostatic water for injection	30 ml (#2)

Blood Pressure Equipment
_____ Manometer
_____ Bulb
_____ Infant latex cuff with Y connector
_____ Infant cuff

_____ Child cuff
_____ Small adult cuff
_____ Large adult cuff

Miscellaneous Equipment
_____ Bandage scissor (1)
_____ "Kelly" hemostats (2)
_____ Needle holder (1)
_____ Scalpel, #11 blade (1)
_____ Pen
_____ Scratch pad
_____ Pen light

Ventilation Drawer
_____ Adult Laerdal resuscitation bag
_____ Child Laerdal resuscitation bag
_____ Oxygen flowmeter with nipple adapter and O_2 tubing

Masks
_____ Premature
_____ Newborn
_____ Infant
_____ Child
_____ Small adult
_____ Medium adult
_____ Large adult
_____ Laerdal pocket mask
_____ Adult partial rebreather
_____ Pediatric partial rebreather

Oral Airways
_____ Size 00
_____ Size 0
_____ Size 1
_____ Size 2
_____ Size 3
_____ Size 4

Nasopharyngeal Airways (1 each)

_____ Size 14	_____ Size 24
_____ Size 16	_____ Size 26
_____ Size 18	_____ Size 28
_____ Size 20	_____ Size 30
_____ Size 22	_____ Size 32

Intubation Kit
_____ Laryngoscope handle with batteries (2)
_____ Adult Magill forceps
_____ Child Magill forceps
_____ Adult stylette
_____ Child stylette

Laryngoscope blades (with light bulbs)
_____ Wis-Forreger, size 1
_____ Wis-Forreger, size 2
_____ Wis-Forreger, size 3
_____ Wis-Forreger, size 4
_____ Miller, size 0
_____ Miller, size 1
_____ Miller, size 3
_____ McIntosh, size 2
_____ McIntosh, size 3

Endotracheal Tube Packet (2 each)
_____ Size 2.5
_____ Size 3
_____ Size 3.5
_____ Size 4
_____ Size 4.5
_____ Size 5
_____ Size 5.5   Uncuffed
_____ Size 6
_____ Size 6.5
_____ Size 7
_____ Size 7.5

_____ Size 5
_____ Size 5.5
_____ Size 6
_____ Size 6.5   Cuffed
_____ Size 7
_____ Size 7.5
_____ K-Y Jelly

Miscellaneous Ventilation Supplies
_____ O$_2$ tubing
_____ Tongue blades (3)
_____ Padded tongue blades (2)

_____ Tape, 1-in, waterproof (1)
_____ Tincture Benzoin
_____ 4-in x 4-in sponges
_____ Trans tracheal airway (#14 Jelco needle attached to 3 cc syringe with 3 mm endotracheal adapter)
_____ Size C batteries (2)
_____ Small laryngoscope light bulbs (2)
_____ Large laryngoscope light bulbs (2)
_____ 5 cc syringe

Suction Equipment
_____ Tapered metal adapters
_____ Yankaner "tonsil suction"
_____ X-ray Gomco suction device
_____ Connecting tubing
_____ 250 ml sterile NaCl

Airway Suction Kits (2 each)
_____ 6 Fr
_____ 8 Fr
_____ 10 Fr
_____ 12 Fr
_____ 14 Fr
_____ 16 Fr

Gastric Suction (1 each)
_____ Salem Sump, size 10 Fr
_____ Salem Sump, size 12 Fr
_____ Salem Sump, size 14 Fr
_____ Salem Sump, size 16 Fr

Feeding Tubes (1 each)
_____ Size 3½ Fr
_____ Size 5 Fr
_____ Size 8 Fr

Injection Drawer

Syringes
_____ Insulin M 100 (3)
_____ 1 cc TB with needle (5)
_____ 3 cc with needle (5)
_____ 3 cc without needle (5)
_____ 5 cc without needle (5)

_____ 10 cc without needle (5)
_____ 20 cc without needle (5)
_____ 60 cc catheter tip (5)

Needles
Straight Metal
_____ 25 ga (8)
_____ 23 ga (8)
_____ 21 ga (8)
_____ 19 ga (8)

Scalp Vein
_____ 25 ga (3)
_____ 23 ga (3)
_____ 21 ga (3)
_____ 19 ga (3)

4-in "Cardiac Needles"
_____ 22 ga (1)
_____ 20 ga (1)

Jelco "Cathlon"
_____ 24 ga (8)
_____ 22 ga (8)
_____ 20 ga (8)
_____ 18 ga (8)
_____ 16 ga (8)
_____ 14 ga (8)

Medicut Cannulae
_____ 22 ga (4)
_____ 20 ga (4)

Ancillary IV Supplies
_____ Tourniquet: wide (1)
_____ Tourniquet: narrow (2)
_____ Alcohol prep sponges (12,
_____ Povidone prep sponges (12)
_____ Safety razor with blade (1)
_____ Waterproof tape, 1 in (2)
_____ Paper tape, 1 in (1)
_____ Transparent adhesive dressings (4)
_____ 4-in x 4-in sponges (1 pkg)
_____ 2-in x 2-in sponges (1 pkg)

_____ ABD (6)
_____ Neosporine antibiotic ointment (3 pkg)
_____ Silk suture 3-0 with needle (2)
_____ Silk suture 4-0 with needle (2)
_____ Sterile cotton balls (2 pkg)

Miscellaneous IV Supplies
_____ Extension tubing 30 in with 2 injection sites (3)
_____ "T connectors": size 5 (4)
_____ 3-way stopcocks (4)
_____ Armboard, 18 in (1)
_____ Armboard, 9 in (2)
_____ Armboard, 5½ in (2)

Bottom Compartment

IV Solutions
_____ D5/Lactated Ringer's 500 cc (1)
_____ D5/Lactated Ringer's 250 cc (1)
_____ D5/2 NaCl 500 cc (1)
_____ D5/2 NaCl 25 cc (1)

Tubing
_____ Administration set with fluid tubing, in-line burette and microdrip (3)
_____ Solution administration set with fluid tubing and macrodrip (2)
_____ Blood administration set with tubing, in-line filter and burette (1)
_____ Blood administration set with tubing, in-line filter and no burette (1)

"Deep Line" Sets and Ancillary Equipment
_____ Scalpel
_____ Arrow pediatric kit (1)
_____ Cook catheter kit 300 (1)
_____ Cook catheter kit 400 (1)
_____ Cook catheter kit 500 (1)
_____ J wire .18 diameter (2)
_____ J wire .21 diameter (2)
_____ Aperture drape: sterile, adhesive, transparent (2)
_____ Sterile towels (1 pkg)

Gloves
_____ Sterile, size 6½ (2)
_____ Sterile, size 7 (2)
_____ Sterile, size 7½ (2)
_____ Sterile, size 8 (2)

Index

Communications in, 199-200
Equipment for, 198
Optimal characteristics of, 194-195
Personnel for, 197-198
Use of, 195
Trauma area, 157-158
Treatment rooms
Adolescent unit, 103
Ambulatory pediatric services, 136
Pediatric unit, 88-89, 92-93
Triage area, 154-156

Ultrasound imaging, 169, 170, 172, 174, 177
United States Department of Health and Human Services, 17, 234
Utility areas, 93-94, 136
Utilization review, 26, 31-32

Vacuum outlets, 238-239
Ventilation, intensive care unit, 236-237
Visiting
By parents, 20, 62, 79, 85, 87
Policy on, 20
Volunteer services, 208-211

X-rays
Chest, 175
Equipment outlets for, 235
Skull, 175
Use of, 169, 173, 176, 177